National Psoriasis Foundation®
This book is published by the National Psoriasis
Foundation, a 501(C)(3) lay, nonprofit organization
dedicated to public education and psoriasis research.

ISBN: 0-9700982-0-0

Disclaimer: All of the information presented in this
book was previously published in an issue of the
Bulletin in the "It Works for Me" column. The information is purely anecdotal and does not represent any
kind of scientific interpretation. The NPF does not
endorse or recommend any treatment regimens, diets,
medications or products, and always advises that you
seek the counsel of a physician before initiating any
treatment for psoriasis or psoriatic arthritis.

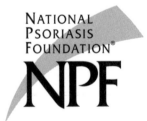

NATIONAL
PSORIASIS
FOUNDATION®
NPF

6600 SW 92nd Ave., Suite 300
Portland, OR 97223
(800) 723-9166
Fax: (503) 245-0626
e-mail: getinfo@npfusa.org
www.psoriasis.org

The Best of
It Works For Me

1991–1999

National Psoriasis Foundation®

What is "It Works for Me"?

You may wonder how *The Best of It Works For Me: 1991–1999* came to be. It is really quite simple—people who have psoriasis want to know what other people who have psoriasis are doing to bring their disease under control. They are on a collective search, because psoriasis has no cure.

In 1991, the National Psoriasis Foundation (NPF) started compiling the fruits of this search—people's tips, tidbits, insights and experiences—in a column called "It Works for Me" in the NPF's national newsletter, the *Bulletin*.

It's a fact that people who have psoriasis learn best from each other, because they share a common experience. Psoriasis is chronic, and people who have it spend an enormous amount of time searching for skin care techniques that bring relief. Plus, individuals do not always react to the same psoriasis treatments in the same manner, and some treatments work for a while and then become ineffective. Frustration and confusion are not unfamiliar to people who have psoriasis.

The best practical advice about treating the disease comes from those who are dealing with its symptoms and those who have years of practice in devising their own homespun skin care regimens. As long as a regimen or suggestion isn't harmful to one's overall well-being, most people are open to making their existence with psoriasis the best it can be.

A recurring column in the *Bulletin* seemed a clearcut choice for publishing the treatment tips and advice people send to the NPF regularly. Thus, with a commitment to a nonjudgmental perspective and an obligation to allow people the freedom to express their treatment preferences, the "It Works for Me" column was born.

Once the column was introduced, it quickly became a favorite feature among readers, and its appeal has never diminished. "It Works for Me" has developed into a constructive avenue for people who have psoriasis to share information—not only about their experiences with traditional treatments, but also their encounters with alternative therapies and the atypical, sometimes unconventional, tactics people employ.

Why publish a book?

The NPF has been publishing "It Works for Me" in the *Bulletin* for nine years. And over time, many NPF members requested that we pool the column's information in one publication. Very likely, this book will be an entertaining trip down memory lane for those members who have been reading, and contributing to, "It Works for Me" since its *Bulletin* debut.

Although we didn't include all the letters we published in the 1990s, we made an effort to re-create the information as completely and as historically accurately as possible. Some reports were omitted because of space and changes in product availability. Still, the following pages are full of treatment ideas and tips that people have shared with us in the last decade.

We hope this information will be of value to you, although we recognize—and you should too—that treatments are unpredictable for individuals. Yet, many practical tips, like moisturizing the skin and using natural sunlight, are recognized as beneficial to most people who have psoriasis.

The NPF recommends that you consult a physician before interrupting a treatment regimen or starting a new psoriasis treatment. Your physician is your best resource for medical advice and guidance in controlling psoriasis.

How to use this book and how to find more information

Keep in mind that some of the products or treatments mentioned in the book may no longer be available, because the book's entries cover nine years. Consult a pharmacist about products that you do not find on the store shelves.

We included contact and ordering information wherever it seemed appropriate. However, for an up-to-date listing of products for psoriasis and psoriatic arthritis, the NPF publishes another resource called the *Product Directory* [call the NPF at (800) 723-9166 for your free copy]. This resource lists information for more than 300 over-the-counter (OTC) and prescription products. Also, the directory may offer more detailed information about products or list other brands with the same ingredients that you read about in *The Best of It Works For Me*. If you still do not find the product you are looking for or an alternative, contact your doctor or pharmacist for suggestions.

The NPF would like to thank everyone who has shared their experiences through the "It Works for Me" column over the past nine years.

It Works for Me

(Note: prior to July '93 no names and/or states were given with the submissions.)

March/April '91

Vaseline and Epsom salts

Applying petrolatum (Vaseline) three times a day and bathing in an Epsom salt solution helps one person who has widespread psoriasis. While bathing, he gently rubs his skin with a "pumice sponge" to peel off dead cells, taking care not to make the skin bleed. (One could substitute any mildly abrasive device, such as the gritty stones used for callus removal.) He said the treatment stopped the cracking of his palms and soles and improved the psoriasis everywhere except the groin and the corners of his eyes. He has continued the treatment for a year and is using no other medicines.

Boric acid, baking soda

Itching went away for a member who dissolved 3 tablespoons of boric acid in 16 ounces of water. Using it on her hands like lotion and soaking her feet in the solution, she would then air dry her skin. No moisturizers were used. At times when her feet and hands were dry and cracked, she mixed boric acid with petrolatum and rubbed it on as needed.

She also dissolved 1 1/2 cups of baking soda in 3 gallons of water and poured the mixture over her body. The solution deodorizes and cleanses the body, she said, and sometimes she simply applied the mixture with a cloth. She let the solution evaporate or air dry.

Household bath oil

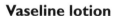

Two teaspoons of olive oil and a large glass of milk added to the bath water is an old remedy called "Sulzberger's household bath oil," according to a dermatology medical textbook. It can make the skin soft (benefit) and the bathtub slippery (risk).

Vaseline lotion

After bathing, one member applies Vaseline Dermatology Formula lotion, leaves it on the skin for a few minutes, then towels vigorously to moisturize the skin and remove scales.

Tar staining

Lestoil, manufactured by Noxell Corporation, removes tar stains from porcelain bathtubs. If porcelain has become thin and porous, the product is less effective. Fiberglass tubs are hardest to keep stain-free.

PUVA nausea

Psoralens are the "P" in PUVA, a combination therapy that makes use of ultraviolet light type A (UVA) to clear psoriasis. But some people experience nausea from taking psoralens and may give up the therapy for that reason.

A Portland, OR, member found that eating instant oatmeal and Pop Tarts curbed the nausea. This became his breakfast each time he was scheduled for a morning PUVA treatment.

Other suggestions from people who had nausea from psoralens: chew gum right after taking the psoralen. Digestive juices keep working and seem to digest the medicine better. Or, divide the day's pills into two portions. Take half of them with food, wait 15 minutes, then take the remainder with food. The 15-minute delay doesn't seem to affect the peak level of the medicine in the body.

May/June '91

Genital psoriasis

The following reports came to NPF in response to a member's plea for practical tips in treating genital psoriasis.

When widespread itching and painful, disfiguring lesions on the penis did not respond to topical medications, one NPF member went from doctor to doctor. After some experimentation, he and one dermatologist discovered that Hytone, a low-potency [prescription] steroid, brought some relief in calming the acute phase of symptoms. (A generic steroid product was not effective, he told NPF.) However, the dermatologist cautioned against using Hytone too frequently because steroids have the potential of thinning the skin.

Next, after studying NPF literature, the man with genital psoriasis decided to try exposure to sunlight—a somewhat difficult undertaking. "It is not easy to get sunlight on genital areas in our prudish society. One can sit in the sun in one's own backyard, if there is one, and the yard is private. Or, you can go where direct sunlight is enjoyed as a matter of course. And that, of course, is a nudist park," he said.

With a daily hour of sunning, the Hytone was needed only once or twice every few weeks. A move to Florida was helpful, since the new home is located near a nudist park.

The member said warm temperature and humidity alone seem to alleviate the itching of his limbs, particularly during vacations in the Caribbean. "In summary, I found real relief in the combination of Hytone and sunshine," he concluded.

For another NPF member, job stress, excess weight and drinking were associated with a flaring of genital psoriasis. A government worker whose job involved inspecting military installations, he spent most of his time "on the road with excessive drinking due to my stress and nothing better to do at night." Prescribed medications did not work.

At the recommendation of a physician who headed a military hospital, the government employee was placed in a desk job where he came home every night and on weekends. He was prescribed 0.05% Cordran [prescription topical steroid] ointment to be applied several times daily.

"After several weeks on the desk job without stress, watching my diet very closely and losing weight, reducing my alcohol consumption to only one drink at night and applying the Cordran, my genital psoriasis disappeared." It returns if he gets stressed or overeats and drinks too much. "After taking necessary precautions and using Cordran, I no longer have a problem with genital psoriasis," he said.

September/October '91

Shampoo soak

Neutrogena T/Gel shampoo brought so much improvement to the scalp and hands of one NPF member, that she added two capfuls to her nightly bath. "I find my psoriasis much improved, no more itching, and with a healthy glow. My dermatologist is very pleased. The most amazing part is that I could never use tar products before. I hope they never discontinue T/Gel shampoo!"

Domeboro powder

A Virginia member says the following treatment "alleviates cracking, and hastens the removal of scales, and soothes the itching" of her foot psoriasis. She dissolves two packets of Domeboro powder [an astringent solution made by Bayer, available over the counter in drugstores] in a quart or two of hot water and soaks for 15-20 minutes. Scales can be removed by pumice stone or other abrasive means. She applies a petrolatum/salicylic emollient. She sometimes covers her feet with plastic film after the treatment. "Sounds like a hair care bake-off recipe, doesn't it?" she says.

Styling gel

Polymeric styling gel and Humectress Moisture Potion by Nexxus made a remarkable difference for a gentleman from New Jersey. He applies the styling gel to the hair and blows it dry. He says the gel has great moisturizing powers, and he finds it stays in the scalp all day. He buys the products at barber shops and retail stores.

Salt and oil bath

At the national psoriasis conference held in Boston, people exchanged home remedies in a workshop on nontraditional treatments. This recipe was described as a psoriasis bath soak.

Fill your bathtub with warm water (not hot). Add 1 cup of Epsom salts, $1/4$ cup Dead Sea salt and a squirt of bath oil (or baby oil). Then soak for at least 15 minutes. Apply oil to the skin immediately after leaving the water.

November/December '91

Anti-nausea tips for PUVA

Dr. J.V.W., M.D., of MA says, "Our office had some success in suggesting soda pop rather than milk in taking Oxsoralen Ultra." He said that people report less nausea with cola drinks.

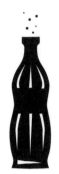

A member from Syracuse, NY, found that taking the psoralen pills with a $1/2$ pint of chocolate milk banished the nausea he had always experienced previously.

Psoriasis and swimming

"For a while I worked at a health spa and part of my job was to teach water aerobics. We all know how a swimming suit strikes terror into the heart of a person with psoriasis, and my legs were in bad shape at the time. My solution was to wear black sports tights over my swimsuit. I told my students that they could see my leg movements under water better that way. They thought it was a brilliant idea. Ha!"

Scalp tips

I have severe scalp psoriasis, and I found that alternating T/Gel Shampoo and Pentrax Shampoo [OTC tar shampoos] has done wonders.

My scalp was helped by L'Oreal Preference and Excellence hair dye. Other brands caused an allergic reaction.

Olive or vegetable oil under a shower cap overnight removes the scales from my scalp.

My ears cleared, and the scaling seems to be controlled (not cured) after using Nizoral Shampoo [OTC dandruff shampoo].

January/February '92

Help for pustular psoriasis

N.H. of CO tells NPF members to never give up hope. A severe case of pustular psoriasis caused the skin on her feet and hands to thicken, crack and bleed. She wore soft slippers, even at work, because shoes caused pain and worsened bleeding.

A physician and a nurse, both practiced in psoriasis care, directed her to soak her feet and hands nightly, then to apply Psorcon ointment [a prescription corticosteroid] to the wet skin. She was instructed to top the Psorcon with a mixture of Purpose Skin Cream and Epilyt (over-the-counter preparations). She then covered her creamed hands and feet with wet gloves and stockings. She topped the wet garments with plastic bags and plastic gloves, wearing these coverings for two hours every night. [Note: Do not occlude a prescription medication unless directed by a physician.]

At bedtime, she rubbed her feet and hands with zinc oxide ointment and wore white cotton stockings to bed. Mornings, she applied more cortisone creams before donning clean stockings.

Three months later, she started the psoralen and ultraviolet A therapy called PUVA, beginning with several treatments a week. She eventually cleared and went to a maintenance schedule of one treatment every few weeks. She still soaks and moisturizes with over-the-counter preparations, but doesn't use the socks and gloves. "I still have some redness, but no fissures, peeling or thick skin," she said.

Her doctor calls it a "miracle." She calls it a reward for hard work. "I use my moisturizers regularly. I cooperate with my doctor and my nurse. This is maintenance, and I will need to do it the rest of my life." By maintaining the treatment, she says, "I am controlling my psoriasis instead of giving my life over to it, as I did when I had so much pain and was nearly disabled."

A Michigan woman with pustular psoriasis on the palms of the hands and one side of one foot found that Oxipor VHC Psoriasis Lotion [an OTC tar product] used with or without a light film of petrolatum was a great help. "If a patch breaks out, I re-apply the solution for a few days. My problem for the most part is gone. I'm glad to share this. I've gone through a lot of expense with prescription and over-the-counter products and was pleased to find something that works."

A San Francisco woman says, "Perseverance, hard work, education and a greasy lifestyle has paid off. I am now 99 percent clear from plaque and erythrodermic psoriasis that once covered 90 percent of my body."

Erythrodermic psoriasis generally appears as a painful, itchy reddening of the skin. The skin sheds fine scales and sometimes comes off in large sheets. The skin's barrier function is compromised, and swelling and infection can result. Often, hospital care is needed.

"When I moved around, my skin cracked and bled. I welcomed the pain as relief to the intense itching," she recalls, wincing at the memory. She said that home UVB therapy, baths with Aveeno products and Virgin Skin soap plus the continuous use of a tar (LCD) and moisturizer (Aquaphor) mixture has made a significant difference.

Aveeno is an over-the-counter oatmeal bath product, and Virgin Skin soap is an enzyme soap said by its maker to help in the removal of dead cells. The tar is Liquor Carbonis Detergens (LCD), a dark liquid that smells like motor oil. Numerous prescription formulas contain LCD, but it can be purchased from a pharmacist without prescription. Aquaphor is an over-the-counter moisturizer.

Ordinarily, a physician will direct a pharmacist to compound LCD and Aquaphor. The NPF member says she saves substantially by making her own mixture, working 40 to 45 milliliters (ml) of LCD into each pound of Aquaphor with a flat knife. She estimates she is creating a 5 – 8 percent tar product. "The Aquaphor is stiff at first, but it softens up. I mix two to three pounds at a time. I could use a hand mixer, I suppose, but with tar, the more utensils you use, the more cleaning you have to do," she told NPF. She prefers Dawn dishwashing liquid for cleanup.

She bathes to soak off scales, which she wipes away with a rough cloth. She pats dry and immediately applies the tar and Aquaphor mixture. Occasionally, she will use a mild cortisone on lesions that seem to be enlarging.

Recovery has been slow, taking a year. "There's nothing real new here except constant care. It takes an incredible amount of time. But I keep it up because pain is a greater motivator than vanity."

March/April '92

Coal tar and moisturizers for itching

An NPF member from Washington, DC, writes, "Each morning, I cleanse the lesions with a coal tar psoriasis shampoo or tar soap and then anoint them with a moisturizer. As a result, itching has gone—is nonexistent and what a blessing!"

Calgon for the bath

A pharmacist advised an NPF member to try a product called "Calgon With Aloe Vera" when bathing. "Though it did not put my psoriasis into remission, I was able to gently rub off some

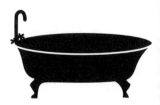

scales after a few treatments, and it left my skin feeling great." The member relaxes in the tub with the Calgon, and then gently pats his skin dry with a towel. "It really helps."

Editor's note: Some time ago, we asked NPF members for tips for the "It Works for Me" column as part of an opinion poll. The following is a sample of what we heard.

Toe tape: "If the toenail is flattening and the edges curl, keep it cut short, and, after a good soak, tape it tightly to the toe to reshape it. It helps!"

"**Water** is what our bodies need. I have a water purifier (Rain-Soft water treatment) in my home which gives me pure natural water—no oils or creams are needed in bath—just white, unscented Dove."

"**Bag Balm** [a moisturizer used for cows udders that can be found at farm supply stores and some drug-stores] removes body scales overnight and feels good too."

"**Oxipor Psoriasis Lotion** [an OTC tar product] applied with a Q-Tip reduces redness and heals lesions. One needs to be consistent and patient."

"**Physical (aerobic) activity** 5–7 times per week helps me."

Natural foods: "Cut out sugar, dairy, red meat, acidic foods; eat only natural, whole foods."

A day at the beach: "Playing in the ocean—nothing beats two days at the beach in sun and salt water for clearing away scales."

"If you see a small red dot that itches, **moisturize** it immediately until it disappears. Catch it when it's young and it may never come back."

"**Preparation H** [OTC hemerrhoid medication] —great for hands and around nails."

"**St. Ives Swiss Formula Vitamin E Lotion** applied immediately after a shower or bath helps. It does not eliminate psoriasis but seems to retard the growth. It is an inexpensive moisturizer as well."

"Use **Crazy Glue** to seal cuts that don't heal."

"**WD-40** helps my arthritis pain temporarily."

"I've used **herbal tea** as a soak, and it helped."

"**Wet packs** on my legs for an hour or two each evening work better than any ointments used."

"**Eucerin** [OTC moisturizer] twice a day keeps it in place."

"**Antidepressants** cleared up my psoriasis."

"Get **pregnant**. I was totally clear for the whole nine months and a few months afterwards."

"**Sun and dry air**—exposure to the western climate improved skin that wasn't even in direct sun."

"**X-Seb-T shampoo** [OTC tar shampoo] left on for 30 minutes then re-shampooed has helped."

"I like a **climatic cure** (living near big water) and using **Crisco** freely."

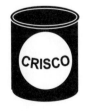

"I found out that **dairy** products and **pork** cause my psoriasis to flare."

"Have **faith** in your doctor and develop a **positive attitude**."

"**Pray**."

May/June '92

Baby oil, jelly combo
For my body, I pour baby oil in the container of petroleum jelly. They blend very nicely to whatever consistency is desired.

Shaved head
When I did PUVA, it was necessary for me to shave my head so the light could get to the scalp. I have never regretted shaving my head. I keep my hair as short as possible because it is so easy to medicate, oil and shampoo the scalp. My wig is such a lifesaver. I can wash my head and in a few minutes it's dry. Put on the wig and I'm ready to go.

Coconut oil conditioner
I have been using Palmer's Coconut Oil Formula (Hair Conditioner with Vitamin E and Pure Lanolin) Et. Browne Drug Co, Inc., Distributor, Englewood Cliffs, NJ 07632 USA [(201) 947-3050]. It has a pleasant smell. I have no scales and my scalp is clean. You don't need coverings, etc. Just apply it—keep it on a day or two—don't put too much on. Then wash your hair. It took one week to see my transformation.

July/August '92

Homemade moisturizer

I would like to submit the following. For about a year, I have been making my own moisturizing cream that I use to treat my extensive psoriasis. The formula and method of manufacture are quite simple and inexpensive.

First of all, I use an emulsifier called Arlacel 83. The manufacturer is ICI Americas Inc., (800) 822-8215. A quart of Arlacel 83 cost me about $30.00 in the spring of 1991, and I was able to purchase it by mail.

I use Arlacel 83 to create an emulsion of petroleum jelly and water. Here's how:

1. In an old coffee can I melt one cup of petroleum jelly over my kitchen stove.

2. I remove the melted petroleum jelly from the flame (be very careful, the melted jelly is very hot).

3. I add one cup of hot water to the melted petroleum jelly.

4. I then add about one quarter cup of Arlacel 83.

5. I mix the ingredients with a wooden paddle until they cool (you can hasten the cooling by placing the metal can in a tub of cool water).

6. What happens next is beautiful. The emulsion cools to a perfect white color that has the consistency of a thick skin cream.

You can try adjusting the proportions of petroleum jelly and Arlacel 83 that you use. The resulting emulsion can have a range of consistencies from very thin and flowing to very thick and solid.

The resulting two cups of skin cream cost me about $1 to make. This has saved me many dollars in skin care expenses, as I use probably two cups of skin cream every week or two.

I was concerned about the safety of using Arlacel 83, so I requested a Material Safety Data Sheet on the substance from its distributor. I quote portions of the Data Sheet:

"A single dose of this product is relatively harmless by ingestion…. No skin irritation or allergic (contact) dermatitis is likely to develop following contact with this material….This product is not likely to be absorbed through the human skin…."

I have been making my own skin cream for about a year and with great success. Sometimes I have scented the cream by mixing it with a drop or two of almond or mint extract.

How did I find out about this stuff? I used to see a dermatologist in Washington, DC, who made his own skin cream. I regularly bought it because it was cheap and I liked the consistency. One day I asked how it was made, and the rest, for me, is a history of savings and a feeling that I have a little more control over my disease.

A final note. I make small batches of my skin cream that last about a month. The manufacture of larger batches (that would last longer) would probably require the addition of a mold inhibitor. I haven't gotten around to finding out what kind of inhibitor I need.

Editor's note: The NPF checked with a pharmacist who said that mold inhibitors may cause skin sensitivity, which, in turn, could cause some people problems. Perhaps it would be more prudent to continue making small amounts of moisturizer to avoid the need to include a mold inhibitor.

Coal tar bath oil

I had to write to tell you of the success my daughter and I have had using "good old" Balnetar [a bath oil containing coal tar]. We've used Balnetar off and on for years, but this time, we tried a different method. We applied it very sparingly, but regularly [directly to the skin], at least once, if not two or three times, a day. I had half-dollar-sized, and larger, areas on my back and on my elbow. Applying Balnetar sparingly also does not stain clothing, and the tar smell is hardly noticeable. We rubbed it in very well. I've had these plaques for about 25 or 30 years—using cortisone cleared them partially, but they would soon flare up again. My daughter had improvement of her psoriasis too.

A&D ointment

A nurse recommended A&D Ointment, and it certainly helps me. It makes my lesions less irritated, less scaly and less red. It is found in the baby department of the drugstores where it is sold for diaper rash. It is much more effective than all the expensive prescription products I have tried.

Dandruff shampoo

I have discovered a shampoo called Kenra Dandruff Shampoo. It has practically eliminated psoriasis on my scalp. It should be used for four to six days and then only once a week as it tends to dry your hair. It does not smell like tar and is moderately priced ($8). I think it can be ordered through the company. I found it through a hairdresser but have never seen it anywhere else. It is really great! Kenra Laboratories, Inc., India-napolis, IN.

January/February '93

Short nails

I have psoriasis under my nails, and they hurt constantly. I see a podiatrist (a physician who treats foot ailments) for my toenails, and as long as the nail is short and "ground down" on top, I have very little pain. I keep my fingernails clipped short, as well. When they get too long, the pain is much worse.

Water repellent cream

For my feet and hands, my pharmacist recommended Kerodex #71 (a barrier cream), a non-greasy, invisible, water-repellent cream, which enables me to swim and do water exercises without excess peeling. I apply two applications on my hands and feet before going into the pool. For bathing, I apply one application. I have had such good results that I want to share this with others. I paid $4.89 plus tax for a 4-oz. tube.

March/April '93

Jamaican vacation

One thing I try to do, if I can afford it, is go to Negril, Jamaica, to sun myself. I think it is cheaper than many places to go, and I try to go in February when it is just warm enough.

Estar and mineral oil for dry skin

Please advise psoriasis suffers that Estar [OTC tar product] is a wonderful product. My legs were in a horrible state, and they are now clearing up. The psoriasis on my arms cleared completely. I also use a lot of plain mineral oil to combat drying of the skin.

May/June '93

Jergens moisturizer

As a loyal NPF member, I must tell of my success. I have been on methotrexate with great satisfaction, but my knees and elbows still gave me problems. After seeing Jergens Advanced Therapy Lotion advertising—"It heals from the inside out"—I decided to try it. I have been using it over three months with great results. I use Aloe & Lanolin and Vitamin E & Lanolin. Both, or either, are great. My knees and elbows are slightly pink with no scales. I use it faithfully morning and night.

Alcohol, witch hazel, castor oil mix

My brother-in-law lives in Las Vegas, and he heard two guys talking about psoriasis, and he told them about me. Well, the old guy told him what he uses, and I thought it's worth a try. There is nothing in it that can harm you. Mix in a squeeze bottle:

4 oz. rubbing alcohol
4 oz. witch hazel
4 oz. castor oil

I use it right after my shower and anytime my skin feels dry. Don't ask me why it works, but it does, and it's cheap.

Soothing bath and occlusion

Psoriasis has affected the soles of my feet for many years. Many doctors have recommended different treatments which have partially helped. However, for the past four months, I have been taking baths at night in reasonably hot water into which I dissolve two good handfuls of Epsom salts. After relaxing, I then lightly slough off the skin with a pumice stone and a good cream soap. Following thorough drying, I apply a good layer of Vaseline, letting it seep well into the skin. Sometimes it is necessary to use plastic wrap secured with a wide elastic bandage to the ankle rather than a clean cotton sock.

In the morning I find the skin is clean, smooth and pliable. The toenails and cuticles benefit from this treatment too. I control the arthritis pain with Advil tablets as directed by my doctor. I am thrilled that instead of always wearing comfortable walking shoes, I can now use my dress shoes once again and have become much more agile and active.

Scalp conditioner loosens scale

I have scalp and body psoriasis. I would like to share some things which have really helped me. I find that the steam room at my athletic club really helps in loosening up the scales on my head, and it allows me to keep scales from building up by combing them out. Also, I use a Queen Helen scalp conditioner [Para Laboratories, (516) 538-4600] every day that has really helped my scalp psoriasis. It has cholesterol and a bunch of other moisturizers in it.

July/August '93

Anthralin stain reduction

I have to use anthralin products and have developed two ways to reduce the staining. At a local restaurant supply store I buy the cheap, throwaway, plastic gloves to use while applying anthralin so my fingers and nails do not get stained. And, when I finish showering, I add some dish washing detergent to the water which seems to break up the greasy, brown residue and leaves the tub cleaner with a minimum of effort.
P.C., *New York*

Murphy's soap removes scale

I can attest to some degree of success using Murphy's Oil Soap; however, I must quickly add that I believe the benefit derived is one of assisting in removing the hard, dry, scaly skin prior to bathing and application of topical creams and/or ointments. In any case it is harmless, I do believe, unless left on the skin for a prolonged period, perhaps.

E.A.B., Louisiana

Water softening system irritation

I have lived in homes supplied by well water three different times over the years and have come to realize how terrible the sodium chloride softening agents are to my skin. I found out from a friend who has very sensitive skin that sodium chloride is not the only choice for conditioning water. Potassium chloride can be substituted in a softening system without any other adjustments, and it is kind to my skin. Perhaps there are others who have softening systems and have never considered the possibility that the sodium salts are aggravating their skin. I hope this will help someone who may also find great relief from a minor adjustment.

C.C., Ohio

Energy pill with gotu kola

I wanted to let my fellow psoriasis sufferers in on something I tried that has been working for me. Of course, I say it's worked for me, but who knows if it would do anyone else any good. It could be all in my mind.

I found an energy pill that had gotu kola as its main ingredient, and I gave it a try. I've been doing everything else exactly the same as before, maybe moisturizing less, so it has to be that pill. It's called

Quick Energy. I guess a lot of those have gotu kola in them. Anyway, it's worth a try.
M.S., Washington

Shaving tips
I found a great "It Works for Me" for shaving my face. 1) Wash your face. 2) Apply Aqualin (a face and body moisturizer). 3) Apply shaving cream gel. 4) Shave.
R.W., California

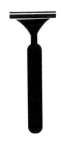

Garlic pills
I found something that completely cleared my psoriasis. Garlic! I started out taking one garlic pill at each meal. It didn't seem to do anything. So, I took two garlic pills with each meal. Lo and behold, I have taken the garlic pills for two months, and my psoriasis is completely healed.
E.B., Illinois

Occlusion for legs
I work in a professional field where suits, dresses and skirts are required, no pants allowed. Having moderate psoriasis on my knees and lower legs creates a problem. Recently, I have been diligently putting on ointment at night followed by Saran Wrap. This has helped reduce the thickness. Then I apply makeup to my psoriasis so that it blends to my natural leg color (or as close as possible). Then, I put on two pairs of nylons. I cut the waistband on the first pair to reduce pressure. I then feel comfortable going out into the business world.
E.M., California

November/December '93

Nail fungus

In a past "It Works for Me" column, someone shared a remedy that included plastic bagging of the feet or hands at night. In our attempts at self-treating, we can cause other problems. Therefore, I send this caution with hope of preventing further problems for those of us desperately searching for a psoriasis solution.

Moist, warm, enclosed areas create ideal conditions for nail fungus! I now have nail fungus which seems to further aggravate my hand psoriasis. Nail fungus treatment is of long duration. This may be the reason the dermatologist recommended white cotton gloves under plastic/latex gloves or foot coverings. Consider this when following fellow psoriasis patients' remedies.

E.P., Florida

Mini-roller to apply lotion

Pay a visit to your trusty paint or hardware store and buy a "mini-roller," about 3 inches wide. You'll find that it will be easy to apply moisturizers to otherwise inaccessible areas of your body.

J.Z, Missouri

Low-fat diet

About a year and a half ago, I decided to go on a low-fat diet to lose a few pounds. I lost about 15. Six months later I realized my hands, elbows, etc., were all cured of the cracks and flakiness I had for years.

For a long time, I thought psoriasis could possibly be the result of a food allergy or the lack of something in the system. I gave up certain foods and supplemented others but to no avail.

The fact I was hooked on chocolate, which is very high in fat, is a major factor in my new diet. I still eat some fat, but I have learned to eat my English muffin with jam, and no butter on my corn, etc.
C.H., Rhode Island

Zinc oxide
I have a UVB light box, which I use regularly and it does a good job on my psoriasis, except for a couple of spots about the size of my hand. These spots continued to get quite crusty. I was using some zinc oxide ointment for another purpose, and I tried some on these spots as well. It immediately stopped the heavy crusting and after about a month the spots are practically smoothed over. The zinc oxide ointment is a standard drugstore item.
L.A.W., Florida

Sunbathing techniques
God bless the sun. When the sun is available, I do the following. I lie under an umbrella, so that my body is in the shade. I only let my legs get hit by the sun. I also turn my back toward the sun so the back of my legs gets sun also. Well, it cleared up my psoriasis. Every day, after my bath, I also use a moisturizer, though I am sure the sun did the trick.
K.A.B., New York

Green Magma and diet
I seem to be getting some help—less inflammation and scaling—by taking one Green Magma tablet with each meal or snack. It is made by Japan Natural Foods Co., Ltd., and is available in most health food stores or by mail order. It seems to be important that it be taken with meals.

Incidentally, I recently determined for myself that Edgar Cayce [Cayce (1877–1945) was a noted psychic] was right about bacon. My nail psoriasis is much improved after I eliminated bacon (and pork) from my diet.

R.W.M., *Missouri*

Shaving and MG217

I've had psoriasis on my legs since 1981 following a skiing accident and a skin graft. I've tried most everything and have had excellent medical care, but the past 3 months have been a miracle for me. My legs have almost cleared following this routine. I use an electric razor on my legs every other day and after my daily shower, I apply MG217 with Jojoba [OTC tar medication], to my legs.

E.A., *Idaho*

Eucerin lotion

I have been using Eucerin Plus [OTC moisturizer] (which is specially formulated for skin conditions that require intense moisturizing) daily for about three months and have seen dramatic improvement.

J.D., *New York*

January/February '94

Witch hazel provides itch relief

I have found immediate relief from itching (caused by psoriasis along the hairline of my scalp and on the back of my neck) by applying witch hazel. It is nondrying and can be applied by soaking cotton in the fluid. Or, for convenience, Dickinson's makes Witch Hazel Pads with Aloe in a jar of 50.

V.B.E., *California*

Editor's note: In an issue of the **Bulletin**, an NPF member asked if anyone knew how to eliminate the mess in applying oils to the skin. Following are responses received from NPF members.

Spray body oils

There are spray body oils available (e.g., Alpha Keri in a non-aerosol spray). Adding bath oil to the bath helps. Pure aloe vera gel seems to help the spread and irritating tingle before an itching attack. Using the aloe vera gel before going to bed helps. One-half cup of baking soda in the bath water and a 10-minute soak help the itching. Plus, a rinse with baby oil and water combination works for me.

E.N., South Dakota

Apply oil with washcloth

Fifteen years ago, my dermatologist suggested that I moisturize, and his instructions were as follows. When finished showering or bathing, wring the water out of the washcloth and pour oil on the cloth, apply to body, and pat dry with bath towel.

B.L.W., Pennsylvania

Spatula/spoon application

I use a kitchen spatula with a rubber spreading edge that is flexible and will not scratch or irritate my skin. Pour oil or lotion from the bottle along the top of your shoulders so it can trickle down the back. Facing away from the bathroom mirror, I hold the spatula in one hand, a hand mirror in the other, which allows me to see my back as I spread the oil, and I can get the entire surface covered with a minimum of contortions. Take off any excess by laying a damp towel over your shoulders and back. For lesions on the back where I need to apply ointment, I use the back side of a long-handled wooden spoon which I initially prepared by smoothing with a Brillo pad. Use the same technique as above to apply the ointment where needed. Rinse off spatula and spoon with very hot water after each use to avoid a buildup of rancid oil.

I am also careful to use a warm, soapy washcloth on my back each time I bathe to avoid a buildup of oil on my skin. I use Eucerin Lotion or Neutrogena Body Oil—either one spreads nicely and feels very good.
M.L., California

March/April '94

Healthy lifestyle
A long time ago a dermatologist recommended: Lots of warm water; lots of exercise; keep weight down; avoid irritation; and, "If canary feathers dipped in mustard helps, Go For It!"
L.R.A., Washington

Mineral oil
I like to moisturize my scalp and the rest of me at the same time. Add one or two tablespoons of mineral oil to a bathtub full of hot water. Then, soak for about 20 minutes, keeping your scalp under water as much as possible.
N.J., New York

Occlusion for soft skin
I apply my prescription salve containing betamethasone (a prescription steroid), salicylic acid (a keratolytic/scale remover), petrolatum (a moisturizer/petroleum jelly) and menthol. Then, I wrap my limbs and body, where possible, in plastic wrap overnight or for eight hours during the day. I also use a local tanning salon

but I don't really know if that helps. I do know the occlusion treatments are doing wonders! I can't tell you how wonderful it is to feel smooth, soft skin again. [Note: do not occlude a prescription medication unless directed by a physician.]
A.J.C., Michigan

Olive oil moisturizer and tar
A non-messy way to apply oil to your skin is to mix a half cup of olive oil in bath water. Even better, apply olive oil and tar (Balnetar) and soak for 15 minutes. My regular moisturizer, which I have used for eight years, is called Kiss My Face, purchased from the health store. It has olive oil, aloe vera, plus other good ingredients, and I apply this after my oil bath. It's all time-consuming but works.
D.M., California

May/June '94

Healthy program
I've developed the following program over a period of 14 years and it has been very successful for me.

- Ride my exercycle for at least one hour every other day;
- Drink six to eight glasses of distilled water per day to flush any impurities from the body;
- Eliminate pork, butter or other high fat foods from my diet;
- Increase my intake of fresh fruits/ vegetables (mostly in raw form) and increase my intake of natural (not synthetic) vitamin/mineral supplements;

- Maintain an ideal weight for my height and build;
- Minimizing stress has also reduced psoriasis outbreaks.

By following this program, I have dramatically reduced psoriasis outbreaks and the medication required to control it. Also, I just reached 40, and yet folks still think I look about 25.
B.F.C., *New York*

Moisturizers, occlusion and a loofah

I would like to tell you what I have wonderful results with, and I no longer need cortisone cream.

1. Vaseline rubbed on to my hands, then Derma Gloves and go to sleep. My hands get the proper oil balance they need.
2. Johnson's brand Baby Bath, very silky.
3. A loofah to rub elbows and heels and remove scales, followed by Alpha Keri Lotion.
4. Biotin pills from health food store. Grow nails long and healthy.

All of the above, plus rubber gloves for working.
M.G., *Michigan*

Cocoa butter lotion and stockings

Moisturizing: Palmer's Cocoa Butter Formula [Et. Browne Drug Company (201) 947-3050] with Vitamin E. It comes in a 3.5-oz. jar. I rub it in well on both legs and then put on a pair of T.E.D. antiembolism stockings, thigh length. The stockings keep the psoriasis moist. I even wear them while sleeping ... especially great for the winter months. This is great for those people who have both legs practically covered with psoriasis.
S.J., *Pennsylvania*

Bag Balm

I recently tried "Bag Balm" ointment on my psoriasis at the recommendation of my husband who heard it mentioned on a radio show as being an excellent treatment. For those of you who don't know what this is (as I didn't), it is an antiseptic ointment used on cows' udders to prevent chapping, abrasions, wind-burn and sunburn. Apparently it has been around for years and can be purchased in a farm and tractor store (for those of you who live in rural communities). I live in a fairly large city (Rochester, NY) and was able to obtain it here in a local farm store. I use it on my elbows at night before bed—it does tend to be fairly greasy so I don't apply it during the day with work clothes on. I have also used it underneath my breasts. For the women out there who have rawness due to psoriasis and bras cutting in, you will welcome this relief. The soreness was literally gone overnight. An added benefit is that it is very cheap.
S.R.S., New York

July/August '94

Smoking, stress, steroids

My psoriasis improved dramatically after I quit smoking! Having attributed my psoriasis to stress, it is quite surpris-ing that the most stressful undertaking of my life (I was a 20-year smoking veteran) would coincide with its relief.

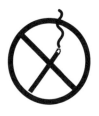

Of course this didn't happen immediately, but the change was evident within three months of my quit-ting. The 45-gram tube of Diprolene Gel [prescription steroid] that I used to go through weekly, now (nine months later) lasts me two months. Even more remarkable is the fact that this occurred over the winter when my psoriasis would usually be its worst.

Perhaps this news will be helpful for anyone considering quitting smoking, but fearful of the added "stress." Incidentally, I had to quit cold turkey; my doctor advised against the patch owing to my sensitive skin!

N.S.W., California

Vaseline

Despite a load of lotions and a trial of ultraviolet light treatments, I remained speckled. Fortunately for me, I had a dermatologist who encouraged me to join the NPF and to continue to experiment with home remedies.

When my back lesions became so irritated that they cracked and bled through my clothing, I slathered Vaseline all over my skin. To my delight, the inflammation subsided and within a couple of weeks, my skin had cleared completely.

Clearly, this isn't the miracle cure, but this home remedy improved the quality of my life.

S.D.C., Connecticut

Sea salt soak

Over the course of time I always found that my week at the beach in the sun and salt water helps the skin. In the winter, I can fake the sun, but the salt water was not transferable. I went to the local pet store and bought sea salt for fish tanks and added that to my bath water for a soak. It helps!

J.J.G., Pennsylvania

Oil and lotion

Because of the NPF, I've become well educated about my skin disease, and am now able to cope with it and educate others. I've tried so many different types of treatments, just like everybody, but I wasn't going to give up until I found one that would work for me. I would like to encourage others to do the same. Here is mine:

Step 1: At the same time every day take a shower.
Step 2: While still wet, rub on Johnson & Johnson baby oil.
Step 3: Dry off with a towel.
Step 4: Rub on Jergens Advanced Therapy Lotion, for extra dry skin.
Step 5: Repeat after every shower, at least twice a day.

This treatment doesn't sound like much, but I've done this for over six months, and it is working for me. *L.J.S, California*

September/October '94

Fruit and bran diet
I eat a variety of fresh fruits every morning and use enough bran and Metamucil to keep bowels loose. No red meat! My only setback was after a steak dinner. Beef is full of toxins. This seems like a miracle to me. *M.U., Florida*

Oxipor lotion
In mild desperation, I decided to try a lotion that I had some success with some years ago. With my wife's help we applied it religiously at least twice a day using cotton balls as directed. The rashes immediately started getting better, and within one and a half months my skin was virtually clear! This has been about eight months ago, and so far there has been no reoccurrence. This is the first summer in many years that I have been able to expose my legs, knees and

elbows without being embarrassed or expecting comments. The product is Oxipor Lotion [OTC tar product]—available over the counter at the pharmacy. Fairly expensive, but worth it! I hope it may be of help to others.
E.T.W., California

Corona—a better balm

I have had psoriasis on the soles of my feet and the palms of my hands. The bottom of my right foot was almost always raw, cracking, scaling, peeling and itching. Before putting on a stocking or sock, I always had to pad my foot with cotton.

After hearing about it from a friend, I first started using Bag Balm, which is purchased from a feed store. This preparation helped more than anything, but did not seem to be very effective in stopping the itching.

About four months ago, I was browsing in a feed store and came across a preparation labeled for use in the treatment of cuts, saddle sores, chapping, scrapes, hoofs and dry skin as related to horses, cattle, small animals and pets. This product is called Corona, a lanolin-rich antiseptic. The active ingredients are lanolin, oxyquinoline, aromatics, beeswax (Yellow Wax), petrolatum and sodium borate water. It is far less greasy than Bag Balm and smells much better.
E.F.C., Texas

November/December '94

OTC moisturizers

Here's what works for me: Vaseline overnight to remove the scales, and then alternating treatments of MG217 Lotion and Oxipor, both over-the-counter tar medications. Be persistent.
S.S-B., Texas

Oat bran and sunshine

I was eating a lot of oat bran and had a terrible outbreak the whole summer of '92. I read in one of my mom's medical books that a doctor had taken his patients off all oat products and milk. I cut out the oats and within two weeks my skin cleared up considerably. I also find sunshine and saltwater help. I go to a tanning bed for half an hour weekly since I moved from Florida to Pennsylvania.
C.B., Pennsylvania

January/February '95

Skin-So-Soft

I want to tell you about Avon's bath oil Skin-So-Soft, both in my bath and as a spray on my psoriasis. It has kept psoriasis in control and prevents itching and scaling. I highly recommend this product for anyone who has psoriasis.
M.G., Kentucky

Apple cider vinegar treatments

I have been tormented by scalp psoriasis for several years and have tried many treatments, which haven't helped. Four months ago I read a paperback called *Bragg Apple Cider Vinegar System* written by Paul Bragg, noted nutritionist and lecturer of yesteryear. He wrote of the malic acid and enzymes in apple cider vinegar that kill the germ responsible for scales and dry crusts on the scalp.

I tried Paul Bragg's formula, and "it works for me." It's not a cure, but the plaques loosen and are removed easily, with the new skin not painful and the itching gone.

Here's the program: Once a day, with a piece of cotton, apply apple cider vinegar solution (2 table-spoons to 1 cup of water) to affected scalp area, patting it on liberally. Allow to dry, and work, for several hours before lifting off plaques, which will be shrunken and come off easily. I buy the apple cider vinegar at the health food store, as it should be raw and unpasteurized. I use distilled water to avoid chemicals.

Each night I use a fine-toothed comb to get rid of loosened flakes and go to bed with an itchless and greaseless head. Such a relief!

Also, I have noticed that regular shampoos (even dandruff shampoos) alleviate the problem only for a very few hours, and then the crust is more solid than ever. I am using Phisohex now, which is an antibacterial cleanser, and my final rinse is four tablespoons of apple cider vinegar in two cups of water. This leaves my scalp clean and relaxed. The next morning, I resume the daily program given above.
V.M., California

Hot water treatment

My son had a rather serious case of psoriasis on the calves of both legs. None of the various treatments seemed to help until two years ago when he acquired a hot tub. After six weeks the psoriasis started to clear. Now, he has been totally clear for about two years. He uses swimming pool chlorine, about three parts per million, in the hot tub water. He maintains the water temperature at 103 to 104 degrees.
C.S., Florida

Inner strength

Here's something that works for me. Whenever I start feeling really blue about having psoriasis, I find some-one, generally a stranger, who has perfect, unblem-

ished skin. Then, I just observe them for a while. They never notice their skin, or touch it, or think about it. They take it with a grain of salt, never realizing things could be quite different. It reminds me of the good old days when my skin was similar. I become more serene just knowing I'm a wiser, stronger person because of living with psoriasis. I feel a silent sense of security knowing I faced a difficult situation and found the strength to persevere.
B.M., Oregon

Olive oil occlusion for scalp

For scalp psoriasis, the doctor recommended I apply pure olive oil to all affected areas and wear a plastic shower cap overnight. The next morning, I wash with Meted [salicylic acid] shampoo twice. When I first started this regimen, I did it for 12 consecutive days. It improved so much I cut the therapy down accordingly and now, 15 months later, I repeat the treatment every 3rd or 4th day. I can wear black once more without ugly flakes on my shoulders. I also use olive oil on my eyelids and ears—anywhere the splotches appear.
L.E., California

MG217 lotion

I am 13 years old, and I have psoriasis all over my body. I want to let people know I found an over-the-counter [tar] cream called MG217 that removes the patches. It is still red, but at least people think it's a sunburn. MG217 comes in shampoo and a cream. I've learned you have to give it a while for it to work.
N.B., New Jersey

March/April '95

T/Sal, cod liver oil, Vaseline

I am a 61-year-old gentleman who has suffered with psoriasis for over 25 years. A friend of mine at work, who works in hazardous waste, was about to throw away a bottle of T/Sal [salicylic acid shampoo made by Neutrogena] shampoo because it was one year old. My company makes fragrances for shampoos and other products. He knew of the problems I've had with my scalp psoriasis and said, "Try this shampoo. You never know. It might work." I had tried T/Gel and other shampoos, but never the T/Sal, as I thought the salicylic acid would burn my scalp. Lo and behold, my scalp started clearing, slowly, but better than before with the use of the other shampoos, prescriptive oils and even olive oil. I rub it in and leave for five minutes.

About this same time, I had a surprise 80th birthday party for my mother, and got to talking with an uncle about my problems with arthritis (probably psoriatic-type). He told me to take cod liver oil every morning to alleviate the pain. I bought a bottle of Squibb cod liver oil capsules and started taking one every morning, along with my high blood pressure pills and Metamucil for constipation.

As of one year and two months since starting all of this, I have one area the size of a pinky fingernail above my right ankle that won't go away and just a little around my ears that the T/Sal keeps clear. The rest of my body is in total remission.

One other tip is to use Vaseline on the body. It costs very little for a 1-lb. jar, and it keeps the skin very moist after a shower.

F.P., *New Jersey*

Radical diet

I am happy to report that I have made some radical, but easy, shifts in my diet in the last month, and my psoriasis virtually disappeared. I have been eating more fresh vegetables and subsequently less meats and canned foods. But mostly, I think it is the addition of many more grains to my diet. I have been cooking a nine-grain cereal about three times a week for breakfast, which consists of whole wheat, oats, barley, rye, corn, rice, soybeans, millet and flax seeds.

With dinner about four times a week, I have been eating a variety of grains with vegetables—brown rice, quinoa, buckwheat, whole beans and tahini, which is made from sesame seeds. Fresh, whole, less-cooked foods, with lots of fiber.

While this may sound very healthy, I still smoke many cigarettes and drink alcohol occasionally. I am a 23-year-old female. I stopped drinking coffee about four months ago, but I don't think it is significant with regards to my psoriasis.

M.R., California

Vitamin D₃, milk

When I shower, I slough off any scaling I might have and just pat myself dry. I then take lotion and slather it on, and on top of that, I put Dovonex [prescription medication] on my bigger patches, and it really flattens and reduces redness in my lesions. When I take a bath, I soak for at least 30 minutes in a vitamin D- and aloe-based bubble bath. The vitamin D in the bath water soaks into my skin, and then afterwards I have the same lotion/Dovonex ritual. Even better results!

I have also in the last couple months stayed away from drinking milk, and my skin, for some reason, just doesn't get worse—even though it's almost winter! I drank 2% milk twice a day all my life, but it started aggravating my stomach a lot so I stopped. Now, my stomach is better, and my psoriasis is not flaring as bad.

K.P., Illinois

T/Gel reduces scaling

I have psoriasis of the scalp and used many products and shampoos, but they were not effective. I read in the *Bulletin* about Neutrogena T/Gel shampoo. It has helped better than others. I still have the scaling in certain areas of the scalp, but it is better than it was. I use oil twice weekly at bedtime, but the T/Gel has helped a great deal.

A.B., New York

May/June '95

Skin-So-Soft, mineral oil and Rex Eme

Having tried virtually all over-the-counter and prescription medications for my scalp psoriasis over the past 12 years, I have finally settled on two over-the-counter treatments. I use Avon Skin-So-Soft; sometimes I dilute it with mineral oil, apply to the scalp with a squirt bottle, cover with a food storage bag, and leave on overnight.

Another item I have been using is one I learned about in the NPF 's *Pharmacy News* called Rex Eme cream [OTC moisturizer]. I use this on the scalp also, with occlusion. It washes out nicely in the morning. I also use Rex Eme for knees and elbows, and it can be used in the groin area safely. I am never without a small sample container for touch-ups, even sunburn.

S.E.E., Ohio

Oxipor at night, Eucerin during the day

About two months ago, I picked up a bottle of Eucerin Plus off the drugstore shelf. I figured it surely could do no harm. Because of the staining, I use Oxipor [OTC tar medication] at night, wearing an old nightgown. During the day I applied Eucerin Plus (either lotion or cream) to my psoriasis-covered body. Immediately, the itching, scales and bleeding ceased. I was so pleased to not be scratching all day, but, much to my surprise, my skin completely healed from psoriasis within weeks.

On the remaining parts of my body, which have no psoriasis, I still maintain a daily treatment of Avon Skin-So-Soft Oil and/or Body Lotion. I'm convinced that the moisturizing has a lot to do with keeping the psoriasis from getting a start.

S.O.K., Pennsylvania

Analgesic gel

I am 35 years old and have pustular psoriasis—the type with severe cracks that bleed if I bend my fingers. Recently, in agony (and I've tried everything, even super glue), I put a product on my cracks that is a miracle. It is Zila Brace Oral Analgesic Gel. It's meant for cuts and sores from braces, dentures, etc. It's in a small tube and is made by Zila Pharmaceuticals, Phoenix, AZ.

It is a hardening, numbing, tar-like substance. It may be unsightly, but it is the best product I've ever found. It holds the crack shut for days.

C.D.H., Indiana

Editor's note: According to Zila Pharmaceuticals, the name of Zila Brace Oral Analgesic Gel has been changed to Zilactin-B. The "B" stands for benzocaine, one of the product ingredients. Zilactin-B is really intended for use in the mouth, and it does have a dark color. But Zila Pharmaceuticals also has a product called Dermaflex which is especially formulated for external use. You may want to try Dermaflex instead of the Zilactin-B. The company says that Dermaflex gel is clear and contains lidocaine instead of benzocaine.

Both lidocaine and benzocaine may cause allergic reactions in some people.

If you can't find these products in your area, you may order from the manufacturer by calling (602) 266-6700 or see www.zila.com.

Nizoral shampoo

After eight years of trying all types of shampoo and creams and using a scale softener at night, my doctor almost gave up on me and my scalp psoriasis.

About three months ago, he prescribed a shampoo called Nizoral. From the first day of using this product, I got almost immediate relief. I started using it every day for one month and then cut back slowly. So far this has been the only relief I have encountered.
A.G., Ohio

Editor's note: Nizoral shampoo is a prescription antifungal product, and your doctor would have to evaluate if you were an appropriate candidate for this medicated shampoo. Nizoral A-D is also available over the counter.

Compeed occlusion tape

I have purchased occlusion tape dressings to use on my feet. I am sure they are good for other parts of the body, but when you walk on it, it becomes sticky and gummy and ruins your hose by adhering to them. I have found one product, however, quite by accident, that works better than anything. It is called "Compeed" [Gruder Healthcare Company, 1395 S. Marietta Parkway, Bldg. 630, Marietta, GA 30067, (800) 654-6558.] It comes in a small plastic box and contains five bandages. WalMart stores here have it. It is about $4 for a package of five. I can wear these bandages for several days. I find if I cover the edges with cloth tape, I have very little problem with the sticky problem. Apparently, it is a new product. I go through several boxes of these a month but they are wonderful for the fissures I get on the soles of my feet.
J.I.S., Oklahoma

July/August '95

Apple a day

I have a dermatologist who always remarks "whatever works" to my suggestions. So, a few weeks ago, I was reading Jean Carper's book called the *Food Pharmacy*. In the chapter concerning the benefits of eating apples, it is mentioned there is a therapeutic result for skin disease caused by a sluggish liver. With nothing to lose, I started eating an apple a day. The results have been amazing. Flaking has disappeared after a couple of weeks and red splotches fading away every day. Previous to all of this, I used UVB treatments and various topical creams that may have helped, but nothing so dramatic as eating an apple. The book says the more apples a day, the greater benefits. As the old rhyme says, "To eat an apple going to bed, will make the doctor beg his bread."

J.H., Pennsylvania

GUNK for bathtub stains

I use crude coal tar in my bath. My bathtub ring rivals any the Cat in the Hat ever made! I clean the tub with no effort. GUNK heavy-duty engine de-greaser.

L.B., Florida

Prescription scalp treatment

I have been tormented by scalp psoriasis for several years, and I have tried many different treatments. First, I shampoo my hair with regular shampoo. Then, the second time I shampoo my hair, I use a prescription of Selenium Sulfide Lotion SUP 2.5 %, 120 cc, leaving it on for five minutes. I shampoo my hair every day or as directed. After the second shampoo, I towel-dry my hair, and use a prescription of Kenalog Spray Triamci-

nolone Acetonide Topical Aerosol USP on the psoriasis
and then style. Hopefully, others will have as good of
luck as me with this treatment.

J.A., Texas

*Editor's note: Other than the regular shampoo used, the medica-
tions mentioned here are prescription. Your doctor would need to
evaluate whether this treatment regimen is appropriate for your
individual case.*

Inspirational reading

I highly recommend two books: *Psycho-Cybernetics* by
Maxwell Malty, M.D., first published in 1960, and *What
To Say When You Talk To Yourself* by Shad Helmstetter.

D.V., California

Diet, vitamins, moisturizer

I have psoriasis on two or three fingers on each hand.
Last January, I read everything I could find regarding
treatments for psoriasis that have worked for some
people. I picked the treatments that made some sense
to me and have followed them for two months now:

- Apply Cuticura [OTC medication] medicated
  ointment followed right away by Resinol [OTC
  medication] medicated ointment before retiring at
  night;
- 400 I.U. of vitamin E supplement two times a day;
- 15 mg of zinc supplement two times a day, with a
  meal;
- Drink a lot of grape juice and eat peaches;
- Apply pure petroleum jelly as a moisturizer during
  the day;
- unprocessed oat bran (about 2 – 3 tablespoons)
  sprinkled on cereal and 12 tablespoons with dinner;
- Cut out meat and sweets from the diet as much as
  possible. No beef, pork, poultry, dairy products;

- Eat many different kinds of vegetables and fruits, and plain almonds (unsalted, not roasted);
- Use Crystal Fine Glycerin soap, vegetable based (in shape of a soap bar), available at the health food store for about 79 cents a bar;
- Take 50 mcg of selenium supplement a day;
- Also, I've been using soy milk instead of cow's milk with cereal.

D.V., California

Apple cider vinegar for the scalp

My psoriasis is in spots all over my body, but the largest and most chronic are on my elbows and knees. I've been using apple cider vinegar in my bath for the past two months, and I can't begin to tell you what a difference it has made. The lesions are getting smaller, and the scales loosen quickly in the water. My scalp is now completely clear. The patches around my nose and in my eyebrows are also gone. And I mean to tell you I'm really "squeaky clean." The itching is gone, and I no longer sit around scratching like a dog with a bad case of fleas. A cup of vinegar a day in my bath is what I do. I don't know that the apple cider vinegar is a cure, but I do know it's not hurting me and has no side effects. It's working for me!

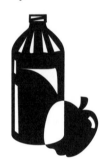

S.S., West Virginia

Rotate medications, occlusion

After many years of battling with psoriasis, I developed two strategies that allow me to keep the upper hand. Strategy number one: Rotate medications/lotions/ointments. I go back and forth between topical steroids and tar preparations, for example. I use one until it seems to be losing effectiveness. Then I switch.

Same goes for moisturizers, I have tried everything from Aloe Vera to Bova Cream (moisturizer for cows with dry teats!). They all work—some better than others—but they need to be rotated.

Strategy number two: occlusion. Occlusion allows increased time of contact, especially with moisturizers (I use lots!), and I hate seeing the counters glistening while my elbows flake due to the moisturizer rubbing off. This can be done at home. I use Saran Wrap with an Ace bandage over the Saran Wrap. Obviously there can be many variations on this theme. There is special impregnated tape, but it is costly, long-term, so I improvised.
D.G., California

September/October '95

Second-hand smoke, itchy scalp, Dovonex
I've gained much from "It Works for Me" over the years and thought it was about time to put in my two, well, er, three cents.

First, I have noticed that my skin rages after an evening of second-hand smoke. An hour or two in a smoky place, and the next day I am suffering.

Second, the best method I have found to calm an itchy scalp is to wear a hat as much of the time as possible, including to bed and especially outside. It helps skin retain moisture and warmth.

Finally, Dovonex [prescription medication] has been extremely effective for me. I am in total remission (knock on wood) in the areas where I have applied it. Until Dovonex, every medication I tried in some way exacerbated my problems and, at best, gave me only temporary relief.
A.S.A., Pennsylvania

Band-Aid and super glue

Quite by accident, I discovered occlusion. I had a crack on my finger (about a quarter of an inch long on the outside of my right index finger) that I had closed with super glue. (My dermatologist gave me an article from one of your *Bulletins* about the use of super glue to close cracks, which worked very nicely.) I put a Band-Aid on the crack and forgot about it for two or three days. When I took the Band-Aid off, the occlusion had taken effect, and the entire area shed all of the plaque that was under the Band-Aid. So I did the same on all of my fingers and it worked so well ... I almost had normal use of my hands, and my sense of touch returned. I was also using a topical steroid medication.

L.R., FPO

Tea tree shampoo

I have had psoriasis for 32 years. About four or five years ago, a hairdresser recommended that I try Tea Tree Shampoo by Paul Mitchell. I had tried everything else, so why not. I've used it ever since.

I now have in my closet one black blazer, one navy blue blazer, one black sweater and one black jersey. When I went out with my husband the other evening, I purposely wore the black sweater. All during the evening I kept asking him if there was any flaking on my shoulders. There wasn't. That is when I realized my head was not itchy.

This product can only be purchased in beauty salons.

B.M., Massachusetts

Apple juice

Many years ago I had a mild case of psoriasis on my elbows. It came and went, but I never tried to figure out why. It didn't bother me, so I didn't do anything about it. Then I noticed that it disappeared when I ate apples and came back when I didn't. So I began drinking apple juice regularly (as the easiest way to ingest apples) and never had a return of the problem on my elbows.

A number of years later (1980) I developed a severe case of psoriasis on my hands. (I don't remember if I had cut down on apple juice at that time.) After several visits to a dermatologist, and the use of various ointments, when there seemed no improvement, I stopped going to the doctor and started drinking large quantities of apple juice. After a short time the psoriasis disappeared, and I've never had a recurrence. I still drink some apple juice every day. This sounds too simple, but so did the drinking of lime juice to prevent scurvy!

G.L.D., New York

November/December '95

Wheat berries make up "psoriasis elixir"

According to my dermatologist, I had the worse case of pustular psoriasis he had ever seen on the palms of my hands. Both palms were almost entirely covered with large, fluid-filled blisters. I could barely cook, bathe, or dress. I drove with my finger tips. I even had difficulty eating. I was in despair. Although ultraviolet light treatments helped, the psoriasis elixir restored my hands to normal. Although I get a few very small blisters from time to time, I can live with those. My normal life has been returned to me. You should notice a change in two to eight weeks.

- Take one and a half pounds of wheat berries (or kernels—purchased at health food store);

- Pour them into a wide-mouthed plastic or glass one-gallon container;
- Cover the wheat berries with one inch of distilled water (the wheat berries will absorb the water; keep pouring until there is one inch of water on top);
- Soak the wheat berries for 24 hours. Leave the container on the counter top. Cover with a lid or paper towel;
- After 24 hours, pour off the distilled water. Be careful that the wheat berries do not escape. The easiest way to pour off the water is to cover the container with a paper towel, secured with a rubber band, and carefully and slowly pour off the water;
- Leave the wheat berries on the counter top for 48 hours. It is best to keep them covered with a paper towel to keep away dust, etc. You can turn the container when you think about it;
- After 48 hours, the wheat berries should have little sprouts on them. If they don't, keep the container out longer;
- Pour one gallon of distilled water into the container. Let the container sit out on the counter top for another two hours, then refrigerate it. Do not remove the sprouted wheat berries;
- After 24 hours in the refrigerator, the elixir is ready to use;
- Drink 6 ounces of the mixture daily (or 16 oz. of elixir/juice mixture, see below);
- You can refill the container with the sprouted wheat berries three more times with distilled water before starting another batch.

Word about taste: The elixir tastes somewhat briny. You may like the natural taste. If you don't, mix one 12-ounce can of orange juice with four 12-ounce cans of the elixir. It tastes just like O.J. You can experiment with other flavors of juices.

H.K., Washington

Ginger curbs nausea

Although I'm not a sufferer of psoriasis but of cutaneous T-cell lymphoma, I have found palliative relief with PUVA. My problem, however, has been the nausea and intolerance of methoxsalen (Oxsoralen-Ultra). I found taking the medication along with Canada Dry Ginger Ale prevented most of my gastrointestinal symptoms. As I understand it, the relief comes from the combination of the carbonated nature of the beverage and also because it may actually contain ginger root, which has been known for centuries to prevent dizziness, as with seasickness. The same effect can be obtained by intake of a capsule of ginger root extract, 100 mg, an hour or two prior to ingesting Oxsoralen.

J.E.B., MD, California

Alternate T/Gel and T/Sal

I hope the procedure I use for psoriasis of my scalp will help others as much as it has me. I shampoo my scalp and hair twice a week. Mid-week, I massage Neutrogena T/Gel [tar] shampoo into my dry hair and scalp thoroughly, cover with a shower cap, and let it "soak in" for two to three hours. Then I shampoo as usual. On the weekend I do the same thing with T/Sal [salicylic acid] shampoo. Leaving the shampoo on the dry scalp for this long period of time has done so much good, and I am almost completely free of the psoriasis at this time.

O.R., Ohio

Cordran occlusion tape

The new prescription tape Cordran on the market is working wonders for me. It is a little difficult to handle very large areas at first. I found using several smaller pieces was the best way to cover larger areas. It is not greasy and is almost invisible and no more expensive than the other topical ointments and gels.
G.F., Florida

Bananas

My entire body became almost completely cleared in a period of about two weeks, and is still clear over four months later, by excluding one item from my diet. That item is bananas, my very favorite fruit. The feeling of being almost clear for the first time in nearly 27 years is unbelievable!
P.B., Washington

Editor's note: Make sure when manipulating your diet, or eliminating or supplementing vitamins, minerals or food groups, you do not harm your overall health.

January/February '96

Mary Kay skin care products

Last year I had psoriasis on my face, forehead and neck. One day a friend told me about Mary Kay skin care products and how they helped her son with his eczema. I arranged to meet with a Mary Kay representative who started me off on the basic skin care kit for dry skin. The kit included a Gentle Cleansing Cream, Moisture Rich Mask, Gentle Action Freshener, Enriched Moisturizer and Day Radiance Cream Foundation. I used the products twice a day for two weeks. In my three months of using Mary Kay, the representative gradually changed some of the products. She changed the cleanser to extra Emollient Cleansing Cream, the moisturizer to Advanced Moisture Renewal Treatment Cream, and added a product to my skin care line, the Extra Emollient Night Cream. By the middle of August, my face, forehead and neck were cleared. To this day I still use Mary Kay. Everyone can't believe how my face looks, and how the Mary Kay helped. Also, the Extra Emollient Night Cream works great on the body, too.

S.P.F., Pennsylvania

Editor's note: Mary Kay Cosmetics are sold by representatives only. To locate a representative look in your yellow pages under cosmetics – retail.

Fortified flax

I am sending you information about fortified flax and psoriasis. My 11-year-old daughter had an outbreak of psoriasis that covered her body. Now, her psoriasis is completely gone and has been for about five months. Her skin feels like silk, and she hasn't had one single spot even after she stopped sunbathing. She is taking no medical treatments at all. No creams, nothing— just fortified flax.

Believe me, I'm not on a mission to bring a negative light on conventional medical treatments or to suggest that they don't work. I'm simply a mother who was desperate for help and found it in flax. I do know that the sunbathing helped my daughter's psoriasis, but the reason I feel certain that the flax helped the most was because after she started taking fortified flax, the psoriasis not only disappeared but her skin was smoother and softer than it had ever been before she had the outbreak.

G. S., Iowa

March/April '96

Soothing bath

Recently, I saw this soothing bath recipe for psoriasis in a magazine.

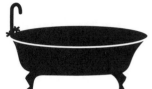

2 cups Dead Sea salts
5 drops bergamot oil
3 drops chamomile oil
3 drops helichrysum oil

Add the ingredients to a tub of warm water. Soak for 30 minutes. Repeat several times a week until symptoms improve, then once a week to maintain results.
S.D., Oregon

Editor's note: Always follow directions carefully for dissolving salts in order to avoid plumbing problems. Oil of bergamot can make skin very sensitive to sunlight and is not recommended for patients undergoing phototherapy with UVB, PUVA or sun exposure. The listed pure essential oils can also be purchased or ordered from your local health food or nutrition store, and Dead Sea salts can be found there as well.

MG217 ointment, oatmeal soap

I am using MG217 ointment [OTC tar medication] that has helped more than any cream used in the past. The great thing about this product is you don't have to have a prescription, and it is not expensive. I apply it at bedtime and it controls most of my lesions. I also use oatmeal soap when I shower, as it seems to soften my skin. My spots on my thighs are almost gone.
D.H., North Carolina

Sock for UVB protection

I bought a full-length UVB body lamp and have found one thing which I have never read about to protect the male genitalia. I cut off the toe of an elastic-topped, fairly heavy, white sock (being sure to cut off the sock near enough the toe for protection) and slip the elastic part next to my body when using the light treatment for my psoriasis.

E.R.W., Oregon

Nail hardener

A suggestion for those who have fingernail involvement: For about three years now I have been applying a nail hardener or base coat plus a hard-wearing nail enamel. My nails are no longer a problem! I have yet to try it on my toenails. They seem so far away!

E.H., Canada

May/June '96

Tar products

I have had a long-standing battle with psoriasis for my entire adult life. During the past 50 years, I have tried everything on the market. I have been a willing guinea pig for all the doctors with new remedies. A year ago, when I was just ready to give up, my doctor gave me a few small samples of Elta-Tar [OTC tar lotion]. I very reluctantly decided to give it a try. My scalp was very bad and I also had lesions on my elbows and legs. I applied the Elta-Tar at night, covering the scalp with a plastic cap. In the mornings, I washed my hair twice with Ivory Liquid followed by Neutrogena T/Gel shampoo. In a few short days I could see improvement, and in a few weeks I was completely clear. My husband's niece also has severe psoriasis. She too had the same miraculous results with Elta-Tar.

N.L.H., Tennessee

Dovonex

Last year I started using Dovonex [prescription medication] ointment on my scalp and body, and within three weeks I was free of scales. I have been in remission since. I now use Dovonex for 10 days each month to remain free of plaques.

The big problem was finding a product that would remove the Dovonex ointment from my hair. After trying many different shampoos and conditioners, I found a product that completely removes all traces of the Dovonex on my scalp, and it only takes one shampooing in the process. I put the Dovonex on my scalp at night. In the mornings I put baby oil (mineral oil) in my hair, comb it through, and rinse it out with plain water. I then shampoo my hair with whatever product I am using at the time. This method has never failed me, and I would like to share this with others.

S.S.V., Florida

July/August, '96

Organic barley

This product has reduced my psoriasis on the palms of my hands by approximately 90 percent. It has helped my skin retain its moisture, which in turn keeps my skin softer. I have been able to stay off of cortisone creams longer than ever before. This product comes in pill and powder form, and it is 100 percent natural with nothing artificial at all. This product is called Barley Green.

A.J.E., II, Florida

Editor's note: Barley Green is an organically grown food produced from young barley leaves. Promoters claim it helps the body balance, cleanse and heal itself.

Starch, petroleum jelly

I take a cup of Argo Starch, put it in my bath water, soak for 15 minutes twice a day. The rest of the time, I keep greased with petroleum jelly.
L.P., Ohio

Apple cider vinegar dip

Your Sept/Oct 1995 issue of the *Bulletin* containing the article on nail psoriasis brought back many memories. My nails were so bad that a dermatologist took one look and said, "You'll lose all your nails!" I tried everything: deep X-ray treatments to painful injections into the nail root. Nothing helped. Then, I discovered the "cure" in a grocery store. My nails are now healthy and completely clear of any sign of psoriasis.

Buy a small bottle of apple cider vinegar. Pour some in a small container that you can dip you finger-nails into each night before going to bed. If you also have it on your toenails, like I did, simply transfer some [of the vinegar] with your finger to them.

Nails grow out very slowly, so don't give up. It works! And what a blessing not to have to hide my awful looking nails anymore.
E.W., Oregon

Replenaderm moisturizer

Last summer, I found Replenaderm [OTC moisturizer] by Jergens. It has worked wonders for me.
D.P., California

Pycnogenol

Although my psoriasis is probably less than 10 percent (of my skin's surface), I'm always trying something different to rid myself of it. The last three months I've been taking pycnogenol—a grape seed skin extract.

Although it [psoriasis] isn't entirely gone, I believe it won't be long, and I will have smooth skin again.
K.B., Massachusetts

Editor's note: Pycnogenol (pronounced pick-nah'-geh-nol) is a nutritional supplement that promoters claim provides longer and healthier life, and maintains or restores a youthful appearance. They claim its action is a result of its being an antioxidant, which protects the body from free radicals. Contact your local health food store for more information.

Lemon bath
I find that if I put 16–20 ounces of lemon juice in a warm bath and soak for 15–20 minutes, my scales come right off, actually, to the touch. My psoriasis is not as bad as some people I read about. It's on my legs, elbows and belly button.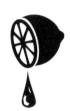
L.T., New York

September/October '96

Aloe and vitamin E
For a couple of years now, my 16-year-old son has had great success treating his once "messy/difficult" scalp psoriasis with nothing but pure combinations of aloe gel and vitamin E gel. His scalp stays clean and clear with a once a week (and less often) application. He usually rubs this onto his scalp at night and in the morning showers with P&S shampoo [salicylic acid] or Pantene Pro V Shampoo & Conditioner in One by Procter and Gamble. (He prefers P&S, but when it doesn't work as well he switches to the Pantene.)

Sometimes he rubs in the gels and goes out—it just looks like a mousse-type product on his hair. The gels hydrate the scalp, and the scales disappear! We especially liked Natural Life's "Vitamin E Gel with Aloe Vera" (because it was all in one) by P. Leiner Nutritional Products, Inc., Torrance, CA 90501. But we can't find it in our area anymore. Now we just buy the large, inexpensive bottles of pure aloe gel and vitamin E gel and mix them with our fingertips and rub into his scalp. It's easy, non-messy, natural, effective and non-greasy.

L.P. and N.P., Oregon

Apple cider vinegar in the shower

In the July/Aug 1995 *Bulletin*, S.S. of West Virginia wrote of the apple cider vinegar helping the scales from psoriasis. I tried this treatment immediately and *it works!* Since I take showers rather than tub baths, I use flat cotton cosmetic pads to wipe the vinegar directly on the skin. Doing this in the tub caused me to almost slip, so now I do this out of the tub on the bath mat. I wipe the vinegar on all my skin to help with any scales. This might be helpful because it "cuts" the soap left on the skin.

J.W., Texas

Sugar

I've had psoriasis for approximately 18–19 years. My father, sister and several cousins and nieces also have it. We've tried a truckload of salves, creams, tars and solutions that dermatologists would prescribe on a "Try it, it might work," basis.

Finally, a niece got a doctor to really analyze her system. He came up with this— stop using any and all sugar! She did. In three months she was clear. She told my sister. She got off all sugar and in three months, she was clear! I didn't pay attention, until a month ago. I was really bad—scaling, bleeding from itching and red. So I finally gave in (I loved my sugar).

Now, three weeks later, I'm almost clear—no more scaling or itching. I've stopped all medication, except "Bag Balm." I am finding that letting go of sugar is a small price to pay for getting relief from this disease.
A.O., Arizona

Scuba diving
I have had psoriasis from the age of eight years old, an inherited thing passed down from my mum and dad. I do find that sun and sea water, etc., work. A new thing I have found is scuba diving 25 meters deep for 20 minutes, which helps to clear it (psoriasis), especially if I do two dives a day for five days.
J.J.M., Australia

Saw palmetto and cranberry
Approximately eight months ago, I heard of saw palmetto, an herb. I started taking it along with cranberry pills and two regular aspirins nightly before retiring. I really had in mind the strengthening of the prostate, with no thought whatsoever to psoriasis. What has happened is beyond belief. As attested to by my wife and doctor, the large patch in the middle of my back is gone with the exception of one very tiny patch about the size of a quarter. The patches on each calf of each leg are totally gone. There is no more itching and the hardness on my elbows and knees has diminished considerably.

I am so pleased to be free from the incessant itch and ugliness of the rashes on my back and legs that I wanted to share this with other people.
R.E.S., Oregon

Editor's note: Saw palmetto and cranberry pills can be found at your local health food or nutrition store.

Jafra Body Silk

Fortunately for me, the condition affected only my legs. More fortunately, even that cleared up with the use of "Jafra Delicate Body Silk," made of silkworms and produced by a California concern called Jafra. Apparently this product is now produced by several firms.

M.E., New York

Editor's note: Jafra products are sold by representatives only. To locate a representative in your area, look in your yellow pages under cosmetics/retail or call (800) 551-2345.

November/December '96

Dovonex vs. light treatment

I have been able to clear myself with six weeks of tar and light treatment at home annually over the past 15 years. I have a home light unit with eight 6-ft. UVB bulbs, two in each corner. Each time my psoriasis comes back, I can control it. When I have to go back to lights, 10–15 percent of my body is covered.

Recently, my doctor suggested Dovonex [prescription medication]. He suggested that I run an experiment using Dovonex on one arm and lights elsewhere. Results were about the same between the two, but I stopped using Dovonex because the cost of my lights was zero and Dovonex was so expensive. You don't need to buy a light booth, though, if you can also maintain yourself with Dovonex. That is my message.

J.L., Illinois

Oatmeal bath and moisturizer

I have pustular psoriasis—25 percent of my body is covered. What helps me is a soothing oatmeal bath treatment (buy the generic; it works better and is $2 less per package) for 20 minutes in warm water, followed by an application of Cetaphil Cream from the jar. This new Cetaphil is a great moisturizer. This allows me a decent night of sleep.

G.R.M., *Massachusetts*

Magnet therapy

I would like to share an experience my 11-year-old daughter has undergone. She has had psoriasis for about four years.

About three months ago we heard about magnets. That's right, magnets! Well, after four years of the battle with trying to clear her psoriasis, she has finally had unbelievable results. We originally heard about the idea from a friend who recommended we use it for pain. I have read that in Japan most families use magnets for many types of ailments. My daughter sleeps on a magnetic mattress pad every night and during the day uses magnetic shoe inserts. This may seem a little silly, but the theory is that by sleeping on magnets or using them on your body, you can increase circulation, which can help the body heal by getting the nutrients where they are needed and getting rid of the waste products that can be toxic to our bodies.

I am convinced that it has helped my daughter. The magnets are completely harmless, and if someone is experiencing achy pain, it may help you with that, too.

L.T., *Maine*

B-complex hair treatment

I have had head or scalp psoriasis horribly for nearly a year. I lost my bangs and hair at my temple line. I have tried changing my diet to one of mostly fish. I took evening primrose oil, fish oils, borage oil and used Dovonex [prescription medication]. You name it.

Finally, in a state of tears while talking to my hairdresser, she recommended B-complex. I went further. At the health food store, I found a product recommended by a knowledgeable clerk called Ultra Hair by Nature's Plus. I stopped everything else. My bangs have grown back, the temples have filled in and my psoriasis is gone. After one month, results started showing.

J.R., California

Growth hormones

My condition is very sensitive to my monthly hormone cycle and has gotten significantly worse since I had a child.

Based upon this fact, I decided to cut out any food from my diet that may have growth hormone additives. This includes any beef, milk and some pork. It's surprising how many toxins are in today's food products. It takes a good month for your system to clean out, but I found a significant reduction in flare-ups and my overall condition. I still eat yogurt to keep up my calcium and call my local suppliers to check for growth hormones in the particular brands.

L.F., California

Vaseline and PUVA

I went to the supermarket and bought a jar of Medicated Vaseline Anti-Bacterial First Aid Petroleum Jelly. It did not put my psoriasis in remission, and I still had red patches, but at least they felt better and I wasn't scaling. A few months later I started PUVA treatments for the first time in my life. My dermatologist and I both believe that the continued use of the Medicated Vaseline and the PUVA made the remission, and most all has disappeared. Thank heavens! It doesn't stain or smell and it stays on without wrapping. Recently, I

recommended the Medicated Vaseline to other friends who have psoriasis, and they have said the same thing.
T.A., Nebraska

Derma-Smoothe oil and occlusion

I have been using Derma-Smoothe F/S Topical Oil [prescription product] now for seven nights and can see 100% improvement. I don't flake all over my clothes, use a clothes brush all day on my shoulders, and claw my head all of the time. It has been like a free gift of a lifetime. The damp head and the shower cap make it work!
O.H.J., Georgia

Ginger snaps for PUVA nausea

I've had psoriasis for 13 years, since the age of 21. I've tried everything, but the best treatment was a trip to Mexico or Hawaii, spending 10 days on the beach.

I was no longer able to take these wonderful trips, so I started PUVA. I have completely cleared after the first month. Taking the psoralen drug makes me a little nauseous, but I just make sure I've eaten before the treatments. If you eat ginger snaps, it curbs the sick feeling.
T.N., California

January/February '97

Soften ointment before use

I am retired from a lengthy career as a pharmacist, and I have had the "heartbreak of psoriasis" for 56 years. As you might imagine, I have used nearly everything available after consultation with my dermatologist. My psoriasis is usually well controlled in the summer (thanks to Mr. Sun and the swimming pool), though I get a few spots in the winter.

A person wrote a while back about transferring Dovonex [prescription medication] from the tube into a jar for ease of use. Generally speaking, it is easier to use creams or ointments directly from the tube to avoid contamination. If the problem is, as I suspect, that cold weather stiffens the substance and makes use difficult, I offer the following: Place the capped tube in slightly warm water from the tap (I use a plastic cup for this purpose). The ointment will have a softened consistency. I use Topicort [prescription steroid] and must follow this method for this product.

C.B.T., Texas

Vitamin E

In the last *Bulletin*, I read a letter from a lady suffering from cracked and bleeding hands. She has my complete sympathy, because I had the problem for three years and no ointments helped. My daughter bought me a bottle of vitamin E oil, and my hands improved on the first application. I used the oil until my hands were completely healed and have never had a problem since.

M.B., Massachusetts

Exorex

I ordered Exorex [tar product] from an ad. I was skeptical, but after only two weeks, I began to clear. Within six weeks I bought my first bathing suit in 10 years. Although I still had some patches on my legs, they were just red, not flaky. Many of the patches have not regained color and are white. But, after years of rough, flaky skin, smooth white spots are OK with me! After about two months of treatment I was able to stop using the product except in a few areas.

S.G.M., California

Derma-Smoothe, tar products

I use Derma-Smoothe F/S Topical oil [prescription medication] on my head the night before shampooing. My hair and scalp are oily so it takes about three shampoos to get my hair squeaky clean. Then I use Grandpa's Tar Soap as a final wash, leaving it on my hair a few minutes before rinsing. Then I gradually work MG217 Dual Treatment [tar] lotion into my scalp, leaving it on at least five to ten minutes (or longer if I can). I rinse it out and set my hair as usual. The Grandpa's Tar Soap, MG217 Dual Treatment and MG217 Ointment are over the counter and not expensive. On my body, I bathe with Grandpa's Tar Soap. I rub a small dab of MG217 Dual Treatment on all the psoriasis places and let it dry. Then I apply MG217 Ointment and let it dry. This way of treating my psoriasis seems to be working fine.

G.L., South Carolina

March/April '97

Laundry tips

I have discovered that the laundry retains a lot of chemicals. For the past two years, I have been using half the detergent recommended, and I rinse the wash a second time after the laundry is finished.

J.F., Florida

Allergic reaction to eyeglasses

I had a real problem with psoriasis on my scalp for around four or five years. About six months ago, I went to order a new pair of glasses. The optometrist said that some people have an allergic reaction to plain steel frames and due to the high alkaline stains on my steel frames, he figured I could be allergic.

I had psoriasis on quite a bit of my scalp. I'd say a good 20 percent, especially around the ears. The doctor suggested I either get stainless steel or titanium frames to maybe stop the allergic reaction. I chose the titanium. I used Dovonex, Temovate [prescription medications] and special shampoos on my scalp for the last four or five years. But since getting titanium frames, presto magic, I now have no psoriasis on my scalp. (Knock on wood.) Sure hope it stays that way.
M.B., Minnesota

Homeopathy

I recently began using homeopathic products to treat my guttate psoriasis, which encompassed nearly 70 percent of my body, with nail and severe scalp involvement. Needless to say, I was miserable watching my body deteriorate before my eyes.

A friend suggested homeopathy. I purchased Dr. Andrew Lockie's book, *The Family Guide to Homeopathy*, and began self-treatment. Since homeopathy is based upon matching remedies to symptoms, this was fairly easy to follow.

It is now two months later, and I am still clear. Even my nails are beginning to grow in normally. Since the principle behind this treatment is that if something is not the right remedy, it won't harm you, it just won't help. Also, it is not designed for constant use—once the right remedy is found and triggers the body's self-healing, it is not necessary to continue to take it.
A.K., Maryland

Salmon diet

I have had psoriasis for over 15 years and tried most of the prescription treatments with very little success. However, recent articles on the benefits of fish oil therapies caused me to change my diet and try salmon.

To date, it has dramatically helped my condition. I take salmon from a can and make a sandwich. I generally eat the sandwiches three to four times a week. The improvement was very quick, within one to two weeks, and I have maintained the improvement for the past two to three months. I had visible psoriasis on my elbow, knee and throughout my scalp. Other than minor flaking and a small lesion now and again, the problem has gone away.

R.H., Iowa

Coffee break

One Friday night, as we were preparing a few songs for a church event, the organist convinced me that avoiding coffee would improve my voice. Saturday I skipped the coffee, and it seemed to help so I decided to abstain for Sunday choir as well. Monday morning at work the coffee can was empty. I decided I would try to kick the habit. I was used to drinking coffee all day long, but went caffeine-free cold turkey.

Within two weeks, my hands were vastly improved, and, except for a couple of very small patches, they have been normal for the past two years. I didn't notice headaches, irritability or other withdrawal symptoms. I now drink only one or two cups of coffee on occasion.

I am not making any claims. This may have been a complete coincidence. But the change was so dramatic, and such a pleasant and long-lasting surprise, that I thought I would share it with you.

R.G., Minnesota

Mahonia aquifolium mixture

I have several small Oregon Grape Holly (Mahonia aquifolium) plants in my yard. I checked in *Rodale's Illustrated Encyclopedia of Herbs*. This revealed that the active ingredient, berberine, was used by the American Indians to treat skin conditions and is still considered by homeopaths to be effective in treating acne, eczema, herpes and psoriasis. It recommended external use of the tincture for these conditions. (The negative side effects were attributed to the internal use of high doses of berberine.) I decided to give it a try.

Following the directions that I found, I added one teaspoon of chopped root-stock to a miniature bottle of gin at room temperature. I let this sit for two weeks, shaking it every few days. The liquid turned a clear yellow.

Once the tincture was ready, I added a tablespoon of it to a moisturizing cream I have been using for about two years. (This cream is a combination of Revco's Vera Dry Skin Cream, plus aloe vera gel and baby oil.) I began applying the lotion to my skin twice a day. The results were amazing. After one week, the lesions on my arms have almost disappeared. Those on my legs are greatly diminished. But the most spectacular results have been on my ears and along my hairline. Also, I had used nothing on my skin for about a month prior to trying this solution.

C.C., *Virginia*

Jergens Skin Care

By using a combination of Jergens Mild Soap and Skin Care Lotion (both are sold at Dollar Stores or your local grocery store), I have been able to obtain relief, a sort of control I never got with expensive medications, and it even caused some new spots of psoriasis to go away.

The Jergens Skin Care Lotion costs $1 per bottle (at Dollar Stores) and is the only one that works. The method to use is wet the soap and work it into a sort of paste. Coat the spots with paste and let dry. Once or twice a day is enough. Just leave it on until you normally wash. At bedtime, coat surfaces with the Skin

Care Lotion, which at this time can be applied right over the dried soap paste.

Particularly itchy spots will be soothed with the soap paste. It also covers face spots so they become less noticeable. On a few angry hurting spots, I also spot with iodine.

R.V., Florida

Suntan

While on an extended work assignment in Singapore in 1979, I spent a lot of time in the hot sun, and it seemingly worked miracles for me. Upon my return to the States, I asked my dermatologist, and he confirmed that the sun was helpful to many patients. When asked about the possible danger from too much sun exposure, he said that he could cure skin cancer but he could not cure psoriasis!

Enough said. I now get all the sun I can, developing a beautiful brown tan each summer with no trace of psoriasis. So for the past 15 years I have not used any messy ointments or anything else—only the sun. Although lesions sometimes appear in late winter (when sun tans are tough to maintain), they clear up as soon as our Texas sun tans me up again!

W.C., Texas

Editor's note: Be aware of your skin type, how much sun it can take and protect uninvolved skin with sunscreens. A sunburn will sometimes cause the Koebner phenomenon. Yearly visits to the dermatologist to check for skin cancer are advised.

May/June '97

Pickle recipe

I have seen many recent ads promoting the healing abilities of natural products such as honey, garlic and vinegar. So I'm sending a recipe involving the latter, which I believe has relieved my psoriasis symptoms! "Can't hurt. Might help," and tastes mighty good:

Country Chunk Pickles
- Drain and rinse 1 qt. jar grocery store dill pickles,
- Slice into chunks and put back in jar.
- Mix ½ cup vinegar, 2¾ cup sugar, ½ cup (or more) hot water until clear. Pour over the chunks to cover.
- Add 1 rounded tablespoon of pickling spice.
- Cap the jar and keep in refrigerator for at least four days, turning often, before serving.
  Enjoy! I also used Dovonex [prescription medication].

R.E., New Mexico

NSAIDs for arthritis, Dovonex, tar and vitamin E for psoriasis

I am a little reluctant to write this because no two people react to the medications in the same way. I have had psoriasis for nearly 40 years, and I've tried many, many different medications. I also have the arthritis to go with it. I have found the nonsteroidal anti-inflammatory drugs (NSAIDs) work differently for different people. I have taken Meclomen (meclofenamate sodium) 100 mg three or four times a day for the last 17 years. It is the only NSAID that works for me.

When Meclomen came out in 1980, there were reports that some psoriatic patients experienced a clearing of the plaques. I did not have such good fortune. I did get relief from the pain and inflammation of the arthritis. However, the joints in my hands, fingers, wrists, knees and ankles have continued to deteriorate due to the disease process. I am very comfortable 99 percent of the time.

Secondly, I have experienced a clearing of the plaques during the past six months. The only thing that I have done differently is add 400 IU of vitamin E to my diet each day. I am not a proponent of vitamin E. I started taking it only to please my wife, who thinks it might have some protective capability against heart attacks. I have been applying a coal tar solution to the plaques after my bath at night.

In the morning I apply Dovonex [prescription medication] to the plaques. I have been using Dovonex for about 2½ years, the coal solution for 15 years. The plaques are gone. My fingernails are clearing up. The pitting is going away—slowly, to be sure. I am not sure what caused this remission, but I am delighted!

Incidentally, I retired after 30 years of service with Parke-Davis (makers of Meclomen).
B.L., Tennessee

P&S Liquid

Many years ago I used P&S Liquid [OTC medicated hair dressing with phenol] for affected areas on my scalp. Just put a little on your finger and rub it in. The liquid is oily, but worked after several applications. I've had almost no recurrence.
P.W., Michigan

A&D Ointment

Recently I used A&D Ointment with zinc, the type used for babies' diaper rash, and found it very sooth-ing and nontoxic. It's important to use the above ointment with the zinc and not just plain A&D.

This is an over-the-counter medication at a reason-able cost, and it spreads easily.
J.W.M., Massachusetts

Massage for stress relief

I am currently in remission and find that stress is the major cause behind my breakouts. My stress reliever is a massage. I have found that since I started receiving

massages at least once a month, my only bad areas now are my nails (toes are the worst), and my knees.
C.P., Michigan

Moisturizing soap
My psoriasis was to the point that I could hardly live with it. Baths weren't helping until I threw out the Zest soap and changed to Oil of Olay.

Bathing with Oil of Olay, using no medicines or creams whatsoever, I saw immediate improvement. Many spots are gone completely. No more flaking or itching, just constant improvement. What works for one doesn't necessarily work for another, but I thought I should write and tell you.
J.S., Nebraska

Cetaphil plus occlusion
I look forward to your magazine for new creams and ointments on the market. I have psoriasis on the palms of my hands and soles of my feet. When I use Cetaphil Cream [OTC moisturizer] twice a day plus plastic wrap at night, I am able to prevent drying, cracking skin.

Cetaphil is fragrance free, has no lanolin or parabens. A plastic grocery bag covered with socks works for plastic wrap. For hands, cut a sandwich bag for fingers and place over your hands and secure with a large rubber band.
J.K., Florida

July/August '97

Doak lotion
I use Doak tar lotion, available over the counter. If it's not in stock, it can be ordered. My scalp was very bad,

and I decided to apply Doak lotion every night for a week. It worked like a miracle.
M.G., California

Emu oil
The only drug that has given me any relief at all has been methotrexate [prescription immunosuppressive drug], although this too has its side effects (I would be sick for four days), and the psoriasis is usually back in several months.

As many sufferers know, the scaling and itching are intolerable. Recently I have found relief. A friend who raises emus suggested I try emu oil. I started applying it twice daily, and it soothes the itching and reduces the scaling and flaking. Although it is not a cure for psoriasis, it improved my skin. I am able to move freely because I no longer have cracking and bleeding skin.
G.C., Louisiana

Cocoa butter and occlusion
I have found that a cocoa butter hand lotion with a high cocoa butter content (one of the top three ingredients), twice a day with an occlusive (Saran) wrapped around my affected areas, does fairly well. It is effective, inexpensive and slow. Dovonex [prescription medication], for me, is effective, but slow and expensive.
J.L., Washington

September/October '97

Turmeric, alcohol abstinence
I began e-mail correspondence with a physician in Jerusalem, Israel, that resulted in my trying the Middle Eastern and Indian spice turmeric—one tablespoon daily. The effects on my psoriasis were nothing short of

miraculous. I had what could be described as "mild" psoriasis—numerous quarter to silver-dollar-sized patches on my legs, trunk, genital area and face, which scaled and bled. I had severe scalp psoriasis with heavy scaling and bleeding. So I decided to try the turmeric, which has been shown to act as an anti-inflammatory and has a not-well-understood effect on metabolism and the immune system.

On this regimen, in six weeks my psoriasis was barely noticeable. In two months it was totally gone! This was during a holiday period of high stress. The only other thing I did—which could be a factor—was abstain totally from alcoholic beverages.

I mixed the awful-tasting spice in tomato juice—thus giving myself a good shot of vitamin C each day. I had had tomato juice as part of my usual diet before. After a while I got used to—even liked—the juice concoction. I had also been taking an aspirin a day—just as a precaution against heart disease and stroke, and noticed some minor bruising that I couldn't account for. I had learned that turmeric is an anti-inflammatory— 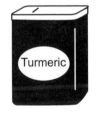 and so is aspirin—so I stopped the aspirin, and the bruises went away.

I was a strong skeptic at first—when you get medical advice on the Internet, you often get what you pay for, which is nothing, or worse. But I later vali-dated many of the claims for the benefits of this spice by searching Medline, a highly regarded worldwide medical database. Most of the documented benefits, however, were related to positive effects on the cardio-vascular system, benefits for diabetics, and possible immune-related retarding of tumor growth.
J.W., via Internet

Editor's note: Turmeric is on the Food and Drug Administration's list of herbs generally regarded as safe. For otherwise healthy, nonpregnant, non-nursing adults who are not taking anticoagulant medications, turmeric is considered safe in amounts typically recommended, 1.5 to 3.0 grams daily. Persons suffering from gallstones or bile duct problems should avoid turmeric.

Hot tar baths

I have been fighting psoriasis for 15 years. I had extreme scaling and cracking on my elbows, underarms, lower back, upper thighs and knees. I tried prescriptions, over-the-counter medications and UV light—nothing really worked.

Then I tried Psoriasin gel [OTC tar medication], Walgreen's Vitamin E cream with A-D-E, aloe vera gel and tar soap baths. I took hot baths using tar soap. After the bath I applied Psoriasin gel first, then Vitamin E cream after each bath. I did this in the morning and in the evening. Within three months all the psoriasis was gone. These products can be purchased over the counter at Walgreen's Drug Stores. Now, I just apply the Vitamin E cream twice daily.
F.H., New York

November/December '97

Honey, vegetable oil soak

About a month ago, I started eating pure honey, a tablespoon in the morning and another at night. It has improved my psoriasis a lot. I don't scale any more, and my skin is returning to normal. I don't know if it is the honey or if my psoriasis just went into remission. The itch is gone, and the scales are about gone.

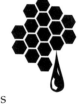

I also soak in the bathtub and put about two ounces of Wesson vegetable oil in, which lubricates my skin. I have been taking massage treatments for about eight years, and it seems to help. This massage thera-

pist is a nationally licensed therapist and recommended by doctors.
H.S., Minnesota

Dandruff shampoo, topical steroid
I have found Head & Shoulders Dry Scalp 2 in 1 shampoo is the only thing that clears my scalp. I cannot believe the results. If I don't use it once a day, just shampooing with it, psoriasis starts breaking out on my scalp. I have learned to shower every day.

I also only use betamethasone ointment [prescription topical steroid] on my skin psoriasis. It keeps it under control. It never goes away completely though.
J.C., South Dakota

Skin-So-Soft Bath Oil
Our family uses Avon Skin-So-Soft Bath Oil to keep the mosquitoes and no-see-ums from biting. This is also good for moisturizing the skin, and it doesn't smell quite so bad. It doesn't take a lot and it really works.
R.F., Oregon

Vaseline lip therapy, Psoriasin gel
I have had psoriasis for two years now, and I don't feel very comfortable with it. However, one thing seems to work fine for me around the ear, the nose and eyebrows: Vaseline Lip Therapy, Advanced SPF 8 Formula.

The ingredients, among others: Vitamin E, D_3, Vitamin A and sunflower seed oil. It only costs around $2. Psoriasin Gel (Alva-Amco Pharmacal, Inc.) with coal tar solution seems to work fine, too, but for a more advanced stage. It really dries and makes the spots disappear. Keep applying, though. They tend to return after two or three weeks without the drug.
Via e-mail

Diet and bathing tips

I alternate Grandpa's Pine Tar soap and Neutrogena T/Gel shampoo [tar product] for one week and Psoriasil Medicated Scalp and Body Wash [OTC salicylic acid product] the next.

The weather has been pleasant enough to allow three or four days a week of 20-minute sunbathing. Petroleum jelly is still my most reliable skin protectant. I have adopted a vegetarian diet for at least five days a week. I limit my dairy products to yogurt and hard cheese no more than twice a week. Of course, ice cream is a treat I deserve.

I have found moderation and flexibility to be the most valuable attitudes to take in treating my psoriasis. It has developed into psoriatic arthritis, which flares with the same unpredictability as my skin. I have added lecithin, cod liver oil, vitamin E and evening primrose oil as dietary supplements. For the first time in 10 years of struggle, I feel that my situation is manageable.

I have found several simple approaches to take to keep my skin lubricated and clean. I discovered loose fitting plastic gloves for working in the kitchen and non-latex gloves for other chores. I work on stress reduction using yoga, and I have finally accepted psoriasis as something that requires daily care just like teeth, diet, rest and exercise. As I take "one day at a time," anything is possible in managing something as unpredictable as psoriatic arthritis.

I share my feelings and experiences with my family and friends when I need help with the frustration or when something works well for the day.
M.B., Maryland

Tazorac® application routine

I don't have 30 minutes to sit around every night waiting for my skin moisturizer to dry before applying

Tazorac® [prescription medication]. I moisturize with LyphaZome Aqua Face and Body Lotion, then using the cool setting of my hairdryer, I dry the area and apply the Tazorac® with a Q-tip. I got best results on the abdomen. Stubborn raised plaques on my shins responded slightly, but will require longer treatment.
A.S., Virginia

January/February '98

Cod liver oil and orange juice
I have found a way to clear up the skin. What you do is mix a tablespoon of emulsified cod liver oil in three ounces of orange juice. You have to drink it three hours after you eat and drink, and then go to bed. Within two months you will start to see a difference.
S.C., New York

Baking soda paste
I wanted to let you know my hands (on the palms) were bad, so I made a paste of baking soda and water. I kept this on my hands for about 30 minutes and then put them in cold water. It cleared my hands and I'm hoping it will stay that way.
G.L., California

Bath mixture, A&D ointment
I read in your newsletter about people bathing in the Dead Sea with some results. I decided to create my own sea in the bath tub. I used the following: Epsom salts, baking soda, olive oil, mineral oil, apple cider vinegar and witch hazel.

After one night of soaking about 10–15 minutes, all scales were removed. After the bath I applied A&D

ointment with zinc. Patches began to disappear. What remained resists itching, flaking or burning for 24–30 hours.

It's best to take a bath daily.

E.W.S., Tennessee

Maxi-Hair treatment

I have had scalp psoriasis for over a year and lost some of my hair. I had gone to three different dermatologists, and my medicine cabinet was full.

J.R. wrote [in Nov/Dec 1996 ***Bulletin*** "IWFM" column] she purchased Ultra Hair by Nature's Plus [dietary supplement] and after taking it for a month, she had seen results and her hair had grown back and her psoriasis was gone. I had tried so many things, I must admit I was a little skeptical, but decided I had nothing to lose. I went to the health food store and asked if they had the Ultra Hair. I was disappointed when the clerk told me they were out but recommended Maxi-Hair by Country Life. I was so desperate I went ahead and bought the Maxi-Hair. Just like J.R., I am amazed at the results. My hair has grown back, and my psoriasis is almost gone.

L.B., Texas

Pagano diet

A while ago another person wrote in the "It Works for Me" column about a book called *Healing Psoriasis: the Natural Alternative* by Dr. John Pagano. I purchased the book and began to follow a few of the ideas given. This has worked extremely well for me.

I realize that the information in the book is based on work done by a psychic [Edgar Cayce] and investigated by a chiropractor, but there are a lot of topics that make sense.

My psoriasis has cleared up about 90 percent. I still have red areas on my body, but there are no flakes and no itching! I have begun to grow hair on my arms again, something that I have not seen since I was 16. That was 17 years ago! Not only that, the book describes a new way to eat (hate calling these things "diets") that has not only helped my skin, but I have also lost 55 pounds on this plan.

J.Z., via e-mail

March/April '98

Knox gelatin for arthritis

In my early 60s, I developed psoriasis and psoriatic arthritis. The skin problems were controllable topically. The arthritis was the real problem. I took 1600 mg of ibuprofen daily to stay mobile. This continued for several years.

Then I heard a presentation by a former veterinarian who became an M.D. He proposed that many of the simple treatments applied to animals are as effective for humans. Among these, he said that arthritis could be treated by taking two envelopes of Knox gelatin (dissolved in hot water) daily. My initial reaction was, "Sure!" But, having been to numerous M.D.s and still taking so many pain killers, I decided, "Why not?"

I started taking the gelatin, but continued the pain killers for about three weeks. When I stopped the medication, my arthritis was gone and has been for a year. I have full mobility, no pain, and feel great. I'm certain the gelatin diet did the job. It may not work for everyone, but several of my friends have gotten the same results and are as amazed (and mobile) as me.

C.H., Texas

Intensified eye moisture for eyelids

I just received the Sept/Oct 1997 issue of the NPF *Bulletin*. On page 8, someone asks about psoriasis on their eyelids. I have that, and I have found "Intensified Eye Moisture" by Neutrogena to be very helpful. It states that it has 12-hour hydration. I use it once a day in the summer and twice a day in the winter.
J.T., Virginia

Acupuncture, Tegrin ointment

I have psoriasis, and none of the ointments that the doctor prescribed for me worked. My husband suggested that I go to a chiropractor. I did, and he used acupuncture as the treatment. After the first visit the itching stopped, and after the fifth visit the spots were gone.

I also started using Tegrin [OTC tar ointment] when I do start to get a new spot, and it also works.
S.D., Illinois

May/June '98

Excessive sugar

I just wanted to share my recent discovery regarding psoriasis.

I was consuming large quantities of sugar (mainly gummy bears and jelly beans), and my psoriasis was worse than it's ever been (thick scales and unstoppable itching). On top of that I had a very cranky and wired baby (from the sugar intake going to him via the breast milk). I put two and two together and stopped all sugar for the sake of my baby and to see if it would have any effect on my psoriasis.

Within two weeks I noticed a dramatic difference in my psoriasis. It was no longer irritated. It was

smooth with no more itching and scales, and, needless to say, I had a happier baby. It has been a little over two months, and my psoriasis is practically gone.
S.A., Florida

Scalp solutions

Clairol puts out a hair color without ammonia. This product will not hurt your scalp. I have had scalp psoriasis now for 12 years and use the product. I also use P&S liquid [OTC medicated hair dressing with phenol] at night with a shower cap, T/Gel shampoo and twice a day Diprolene (it comes in cream or gel-liquid and is a prescription steroid). P&S is great for the outer ear. Apply it, a few hours later wash it off.
C.T., New York

Vitamin E and occlusion

I recalled reading a letter (***Bulletin***, Jan/Feb 1997) from a lady who had gotten good results using vitamin E oil, and decided to try it. Almost immediately, my hands began to clear, and my elbows are completely clear. Plaques still form on my hands, but they are more pliable, no longer crack and bleed constantly, and are much easier to live with.

I use "industrial strength" vitamin E oil (28,000 units per ounce), applying it once a day at bedtime. Since it is extremely gooey, I wear white cotton cosmetic gloves to bed. It has been four months now, and my hands are the best they have been for years. Even if it doesn't last, I will at least have gotten a break from prescription medications and may find them effective again when I have to go back to them.
L.C., via e-mail

Folic acid

Back in December 1996 when I had my annual physical, my internist determined I had a folic acid deficiency. He prescribed a supplement, which I took for 90 days. After re-testing, the level was normal. I had been on topical steroids only. During the supplements of folic acid, my skin became remarkably better, and I discontinued the topicals. I purchased a folic acid supplement over the counter and continued taking at least 800 mcg/day. Having had psoriasis at least 18 years, this has been no less than a miracle! All I use now is Curel lotion [moisturizer], two to three times a day all over, and a vitamin E lotion on my face. At age 45, I actually wore no make-up on vacation.
L.M.P., Georgia

Rotate medications, healthy lifestyle

I was diagnosed with psoriasis nearly 20 years ago. The doctors and I have managed my severe psoriasis with rotating treatments of PUVA, methotrexate and Tegison [prescription medication replaced by Soriatane]. I also must use topical solutions (such as Topicort [prescription steroid]) to help with those areas not controlled by these treatments.

I have learned how important it is to take very good care of yourself. In addition to regular exercise (I walk two miles a day and ride our horses) and a healthy diet, I spend time each day taking care of my skin. Two products that have really helped me (not medicated) are Unscented Mapo Bath Oil by Herald Pharmacal, Inc., and Aqua Care Therapeutic Lotion with 10% Urea by Menley & James Laboratories, Inc. I use these products daily and rely on them to keep me comfortable and help prevent flares.
P.A.F., Virginia

Soriatane

My wife suffered from psoriasis for over 20 years and tried everything known. The psoriasis exploded over her entire body, from neck to knees, both front and back. Three weeks ago the doctor prescribed Soriatane (acitretin), made by Roche Laboratories in Nutley, N.J. The results have been unbelievable, great. All skin is now clear of flakes, and she has started to have normal-colored skin in patches all over her body. It seems to be the best treatment we have used.
C.D.E., Texas (via e-mail)

Vaseline relieves Tazorac®-associated itching

I was disturbed to read in your March 1998 *Pharmacy News* that some users of Tazorac® were enduring itching. As soon as it was available, I began to use this product, and while results have been agonizingly slow, there is improvement in every area of lesions, and some of them have disappeared completely. The redness that accompanies the use of Tazorac® is slowly fading.

At about the same time I began the Tazorac® applications, I also began using Vaseline's Dual Action with alpha hydroxy. The use was intended to alleviate scaling and proved to be a great success. The itching also disappeared. The affected areas are smooth, and the skin feels pleasant to the touch. There is no visible effect on clothing, even if it immediately comes in contact with the application. The use of alpha hydroxy before shampooing may also help alleviate scaling on the scalp.
M.B., Florida

Editors' note: Some dermatologists advise that the combination of Tazorac® and moisturizers with alpha hydroxy acids may be irritating.

Vicks Vapo-Rub and olive oil for nails

I have found that by applying Vick's Vapo-Rub ointment twice daily, morning and bedtime, to nails afflicted with psoriasis and/or a fungus has cured all of my finger and toe nails, except for three that were severely afflicted. Those three are slowly improving. Improvement was seen within the first two weeks of treatment. I was not able to tolerate prescribed fungal medications, and prescription medications for psoriatic nails did not help. Also, applying olive oil to my feet and hands at bedtime has completely cleared the skin.

E.V., Ohio

Lotion and shampoo scalp treatments

I have had psoriasis, limited to the scalp, since childhood. The doctor gave me a prescription for a coal tar medicine and hyrdrocortisone. For 30-plus years, I have used that, but all it really ever did was keep it from getting worse. One time when I was out of medication, I decided to use hand lotion on my scalp to at least keep it from hurting so bad. After a course of experimentation, I have found that this is helping me more than prescription medication ever did. Every night I shampoo using T/Gel shampoo, followed by Citre-Shine shampoo and Citre-Shine cream rinse. I leave each of these on for a few minutes before rinsing out. Then I use St. Ives Swiss Formula Vitamin E hand lotion, reapplied as needed.

Over a period of a few weeks, my small sores disappeared, the medium sores became small ones and the big ones became medium-sized. Whenever a sore threatens to develop, I start the hand lotion treatment on it and within a few days, it has completely disappeared. The nice thing about this regimen is that everything is available over the counter, doesn't leave

an unpleasant smell and won't do anything to the unaffected skin.
J.E., Iowa

July/August '98

Oatmeal soak

I am a 76-year-old man with psoriasis all over my body. My face and head have been okay. "It Works for Me," as good as anything, to take a bath in Avalon Clear Oatmeal Anti-Itch Bath Soak (Oil Free Bath Soak). It soothes and moisturizes dry itchy sensitive skin. It's dermatologist-recommended and is sold by Cooper Labs. I am also using Diprolene [a prescription topical steroid medication].
J.T., Iowa

Apple cider vinegar, witch hazel treatments

The following treatment has helped me a lot. My lesions haven't cleared yet, but they are smooth and pale, and I'm using much lower-strength topical steroids. I also got this effect during cold dry weather, which is usually bad skin time.

Supplies: apple cider vinegar, witch hazel and a mild prescription steroid (like Desowen). Time it takes (daily): about 3 minutes. How long before improvement: 2–3 days.

Mornings: Shower normally and wash with mild soap. After rinsing, rub the lesions with a weak apple cider vinegar solution (I eyeball it at about 7 parts water to 1 part vinegar). Rinse again and turn off the shower. While still wet, splash some witch hazel on the lesions. Rub gently. Towel dry gently (I find I can then skip a moisturizer, even in cold weather). Apply a mild topical steroid (like Desowen) to the lesions.

Before Bed: Gently rub the lesions with witch hazel on a cotton ball. Apply the mild steroid.

That's it. It's cheap, readily available, not distasteful and, best of all, not time-consuming.

J.R., Washington, D.C.

Porter's Lotion

I've had scalp psoriasis for 50 years. Virtually every evening of this half century, I've spent hours scratching away at my scalp with a comb in an effort to battle the severe itching. I was recently introduced to a product that instantly caused the itching to cease upon application. It is called Porter's Lotion, and it is sold by Gallatin River Products, Inc. The ingredients of this product are water, witch hazel, glycerin, alcohol, greensoap, ammonium carbonate, camphor and rosemary oil.

I cannot comment on the long-term use of this product for a "cure" of the psoriatic scalp, but it certainly works when you put it on.

R.K.B., MD, New York

Topical steroid control

I use Elocon 0.1% for my ears and other private parts, and Psorcon 0.05% for the rest of my extremities. I wash every morning and night with CVS bath oil and Dove soap. Apply my medication twice a day, and when it looks improved, I use Lubriderm cream.

V.M., Massachusetts

Editors' note: Elocon and Psorcon are prescription topical steroid medications.

Psorelief

Recently I found a new product on the market that helped me a great deal. It relieved the itching and started to clear up the psoriasis. It is called "Psorelief" [salicylic acid 2%], and the patented formula came

from Europe from some doctors who originated the formula.
E.S., Nebraska

Editor's note: Psorelief products are available by calling (800) 822-4320.

Tomatoes

This past summer my skin has almost cleared. The only thing that I have done differently is eat lots of vine-ripened tomatoes.
A.W., Montana

Mane & Tail shampoo

It is my interest to share knowledge of a product that has worked well for me. I have a mild to moderate psoriasis condition on my arms and legs that is more of an aesthetic problem than a functional problem. My scalp, however, was a different problem. It itched constantly, and almost any head movement produced a "snowfall" of dandruff. Certain coal tar shampoos helped but always became ineffective in less than a year.

About three years ago, an acquaintance I met at a stock car race advised me to try Mane & Tail Shampoo, which I purchased at WalMart in the pet section. My scalp has not itched, nor any dandruff, since that time.
W.J.M., DDS, Florida

Cyclosporine

I have had severe plaque psoriasis for over two years. I have it pretty much everywhere, including my scalp. After having tried all the over-the-counter and physician-prescribed therapies, I didn't seem to be getting anywhere. My dermatologist then suggested I try the cyclosporine oral treatment.

I began taking Neoral [brand name of cyclosporine]. Today I can honestly say it has worked

---

miracles for me. My scalp and stomach are completely clear, and the rest of my body is well on its way to healing, also. One can't stay on cyclosporine because, in the long run, it can compromise the kidneys. But you are closely monitored with regular blood tests for creatinine levels. The cyclosporine therapy is supposed to be used in a "cyclical" manner, in that when you take a "break" after a time determined by your doctor, it is suggested that you use an alternative treatment, such as PUVA. This may not work for everyone, but to me it's been a blessing.

E.R., California

Editor's note: Neoral (cyclosporine) is an oral drug that can cause a rapid and dramatic clearing of lesions for people who have severe psoriasis, but it is not for everyone. Neoral is used to treat adults who have extensive and/or disabling recalcitrant plaque psoriasis. Appropriate candidates for Neoral therapy are patients who failed to respond to at least one other systemic therapy, or they are patients for whom other systemic therapies, such as acitretin or methotrexate, are contraindicated or intolerable.

Crisco

What works for me is:

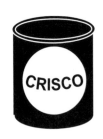

1. Crisco as a moisturizer. It has no petroleum or mineral oil, both of which I am sensitive to. I whip my favorite cologne into it, which is nice, and I keep it in a pretty moisturizer jar.

2. I use thin panty liners to pad the top elastic of panties and the bottom band on bras. They make it possible to medicate lesions without staining clothes and lessens the pain from the elastic.

L.B., California

November/December '98

Nioxin hair products

I have had to contend with scalp psoriasis since my early teens. I am now 37.

About six months ago, a friend, who is also a hair stylist, recommended that I try the Nioxin line of hair products, thinking that it would improve the strength of my hair and reduce hair loss. It worked and, more importantly, I have experienced an almost total elimination of my psoriasis. The improvement is truly astounding, way beyond anything else that I've ever tried. I may still notice a very light trace on one or two days each month, but in the remainder of the month I have no buildup or trace of psoriasis anywhere on my scalp.

This Nioxin stuff consists of a shampoo, a scalp conditioner and a clear liquid product that is applied after towel drying. The effect that it had on my scalp buildup became apparent after only about three to four days of use. Total clearing of buildup was achieved in about two to three weeks time and has remained that way ever since.

J.A., Wisconsin

Editors' note: Nioxin Laboratories, based in Atlanta, GA, produces a line of products including shampoo, conditioner, hair reconstruction therapy and scalp management spray. Nioxin products are available at beauty supply stores and hair salons throughout the United States, or contact the company directly at (800) 789-9617.

Natural arthritis treatment

I wanted to let people in on what I have learned from different sources. I have psoriatic arthritis presently in my hip, feet and ankles (though I think that it is spreading). I take 200 milligrams each evening of primrose oil (four pills) and flax seed oil (two pills) daily. Both of these oils are available in pill form, which I would recommend. The oils have also helped my psoriasis by thinning the plaques considerably.

I also no longer eat red meat, pork, ham, tomato, eggplant, green pepper or white potato. It is easier than it sounds. I have heard about these foods from arthritis groups. Since I have stopped eating them, I can really feel it when I do (even a bite of hamburger swells my arthritis).

Regular exercise has also helped, even though it is tough to do on some days. These simple things have really made a huge difference in my life. I actually forget about my psoriatic arthritis some days now.
L.T., Virginia

Cod liver oil

I have been trying various treatments for psoriasis for over 40 years. Recently I received information on the ingestion of cod liver oil as a remedy. I was skeptical. Deciding that I had nothing to lose, I began a daily regimen of one tablespoon of cod liver oil in the morning and another in the evening. Gradually, after about a week to 10 days, the scales stopped forming. Within three weeks, my legs, which had been heavily encrusted, began to clear up. I am not cured, but I am no longer embarrassed to wear shorts in public.

I continue to take the cod liver oil. This was not a controlled study. It is only one instance but since the treatment is, except for the nasty taste of the oil (I use the flavored kind), so unintrusive and inexpensive, I feel that others who are afflicted with psoriasis deserve to hear about this treatment.
W.P.O., California

Vitamin moisturizer

As we all know, moisturizing is very important for psoriasis sufferers. I've found the best moisturizer for me. It's made by Vitamin Specialties (800-365-8482). The product is called Vitamin Skin Supplement Formula 426. It has vitamins A, D and E in it that can't hurt. It also has a pleasant fragrance. I use it in conjunction with other prescription medication.
K.O., Pennsylvania

January/February '99

Yeast mixture

I have used active dry yeast to clear my skin of flare-ups. It works in two to five days, faster than any product I have ever used. I simply mix a little yeast with just enough warm water to make a thin, smooth paste and apply it several times daily. It's easy. It's cheap (about $4 for one pound in health food stores), and it works for me!
C.C., Oregon

Editor's note: Some people say avoiding yeast in their diet is beneficial. The benefit of topical yeast is unpredictable, according to the NPF's medical editors.

Latex occlusion suit

I have always preferred using natural instead of synthetic products when available. Thus, I could never become enthusiastic about using a vinyl occlusion suit and scouted around to see whether something better is available. I am glad to report that I found a source in the U.K. Sealwear Ltd. (Regent Chambers, 15 Westover Road, Bournemouth, BH1 2BY).

This company manufactures all kinds of latex clothing and was able to make the desired pants and shirt for me. I tolerate latex with no adverse effect to my skin; however, I was cautioned by the manufacturer not to use their products in conjunction with any ointment containing Vaseline or other petroleum derivatives.

J.S., *New York*

Editor's note: Be aware that there are increasing reports of allergies to latex.

Working Hands Crème

I would like to tell you of a product I discovered this past fall, which has helped a patch of psoriasis on my right hand and ankle considerably.

This marvelous cream has smoothed my skin and turned it a faint pink instead of the raised plaques and ugly red it has been for many years. Amazingly, this product was developed by a fellow Oregonian, pharmacist Tara Broadbent (P.O. Box 216, Joseph, OR 97846, 800-275-2718). Tara's development is called Working Hands Crème and, in my case, seems to have exceptional healing benefits.

J.C.F., *Montana*

Absorbase

Due to a job cleaning out a deceased person's house, I came across three large jars of Absorbase. All expired, but decided to try it! Shock and amazement, it worked. I wrote the company, and their response was that they get hundreds of letters like mine. For no prescription and $8.50 per jar, and no doctor visit or senseless waste of time, my hand, elbows, knees and feet are itch free and whole. One hand is perfect, and the other areas are without the usual problems.

S.G., *California*

Exercise for arthritis

I have psoriatic arthritis. I would like to recommend Jazzercise to your readers for arthritis. Jazzercise is great because it can be varied to be as low impact or as high impact as you need, and all the instructors are very knowledgeable about ways to adjust each exercise to the individual's needs, whether those needs include a sore back, tender knees, etc. I always knew that keeping my body in shape was a good thing just to keep healthy, but after that nasty attack of arthritis in my joints, I know just how important it is to stay healthy.

I learned a lot from reading the book, "Toughness Training For Life," by James E. Loehr, Ed.D., which discusses the benefits of exercise for the mind, body and immune system. The only negative (or neutral) comment about exercise is that it doesn't seem to have any effect on the psoriasis itself, but fortunately my psoriasis is mostly limited to the scalp and can be controlled, somewhat, by cortisone.

D.M., Maryland

Editor's note: If you have psoriatic arthritis and plan to start this or any other exercise program, consult with your physician first.

Topical steroids, tar, DermaNail

I have had mild psoriasis for over 30 years, mostly on my elbows, hips and other limited areas. However, I've had a lot of scalp problems and fingernails that were always flaking and breaking. Recently, I found a dermatologist who has helped me dramatically in several areas. The first was on my skin. The doctor injected triamcinolone (injectable Kenalog) directly into the elbow area and other areas this past April. The areas cleared up in a week or so and as of December are still psoriasis free.

As for the nails, he put me on a twice a day application to the cuticle area of "DermaNail" by Summers Labs. It takes at least six weeks to really see results and also apparently needs to be used on a permanent basis. I am very pleased with the results—the nails are

stronger now and are not peeling. They also grow back much faster when they do break. The doctor also put me on a biotin supplement. I'm taking two 300 mcg tabs a day for nails and scalp. This is available at drug and health food stores. I also shampoo with a tar soap shampoo, and this keeps my scalp fairly clear.
P.R., Pennsylvania

Eucerin shower therapy

My dermatologist recommended Eucerin lotion. I find their "shower therapy" works great for removing skin scales. I also use it as a shampoo occasionally.
A.C., California

March/April '99

Antibacterial soap, vinegar for the bath

I am 44 years old. I've had psoriasis since I was 13. I have used all of the ointments and UVB treatments that my skin doctor has prescribed. Recently, I have tried an approach suggested by articles in the NPF newsletter.

I bathe in antibacterial liquid soap, then soak in the tub with a cup of vinegar added; this removes any scales. Then I apply Bag Balm, which I bought at the local feed store. Bag Balm itself feels better than other moisturizers that I have used. I am covered about 75 percent of my body, and all the other medicines have lost their effectiveness. But this is starting to work, really! Bag Balm contains an antiseptic.
D.F., via e-mail

MG217

I've had really good results with a coal tar-based product called MG217 ointment, distributed by Triton

Consumer Products in Arlington Heights, IL. Although I have rather mild psoriasis, I've found this inexpensive product as effective as anything prescribed by my dermatologist.

B.N., Oregon

Zim's Crack Creme with occlusion

I found a hand lotion on the market that works fairly well. It's Zim's Crack Creme, and it's $6 at Payless/Rite Aide. Saran Wrap is necessary for it to be effective. I found it in the first aid section.

J.L., Washington

Editor's note: For more information about this product, call (800) 319-2225 or visit www.crackcreme.com.

Mineral oil for the scalp

I have tried mineral oil on my scalp, covered by a shower cap or a warm towel. This has been very helpful in removing scales.

H.G., New York

Dovonex solution for nails

I have severe psoriasis on my big toe nails, and it has begun spreading to the other toes slowly. The result of this is quite painful. I have to be very careful when I purchase shoes because of the pain. I tend to walk a little strangely and have worn holes in odd places of the shoes themselves.

About a year ago, I asked my dermatologist what I could do for the nails. She suggested that I try the prescription medication, Dovonex solution. I applied it twice daily to the nails, and within one week the pain subsided. Within three weeks there was a noticeable difference in the appearance of my nails.

Unfortunately, I lost my insurance because of a job change and wasn't able to afford the solution. I did have four tubes of Dovonex ointment and decided to try and see how that worked. The results were not as amazing compared to the solution, but I did experience a decrease in the pain and thickness of the nails.

I have continued to use the ointment on my toes twice a day. I apply it at the base, on top, and in the front of the nail. As the ointment can make the nails soft and susceptible to ripping, I use it sparingly.
C.P., via e-mail

Sunless tanning
I just wanted to share a treatment that I have stumbled upon. In the summer I like my skin to appear tan, although I know the sun is not great for you. I do, however, know the benefits of the sun for psoriasis. I just choose not to expose myself to skin cancer.

Anyway, I started using Lancome Soleil self-tanning lotion, and my psoriasis has almost disappeared. At a mere $21 a bottle, I feel it is a steal compared to other treatments, which I have tried for more money and with less than satisfactory results. I hope this can be useful to others.
S.S., Oregon

Editor's note: Lancome products are available at most major department stores. For more information or for a store in your area, contact Lancome at (800) 526-2663.

Dermazinc Spray for genital psoriasis
I used Dermazinc Spray [OTC zinc pyrithione product] to get rid of my psoriasis on my buttocks and groin area. After two applications, I started to notice that the redness of the skin began to whiten and the surface of the afflicted area became smooth. The itching stopped, and a few applications later, everything cleared up. I feel like a new human being.
V.C., Florida

Topical steroid for genital area

Occasionally, I am afflicted by psoriasis of the genital area. The area involved is my groin. My dermatologist prescribed Lidex. Lidex is also available in generic form under the name of fluocinonide. This medication is to be applied every day as needed. A good moisturizer on the off days is also helpful. This has done the trick for me, and I hope it will be helpful to others with this problem.

H.S., Ohio

Editor's note: Be careful when using any topical steroid, particularly those as strong as or stronger than Lidex, in the genital area. Skin in this area is very sensitive to steroids and more likely to develop steroid side effects, such as stretch marks and atrophy.

Estrogen replacement therapy

I am a white woman, age 64, and have had psoriasis on my legs and elbows. I was also suffering greatly in the genital area. My psoriasis came on in my 50s, coinciding with menopause. I was taking Estrace [estrogen replacement therapy] (1 mg daily) and Provera (5.0 mg daily) at the time. When my gynecologist cut my Provera in half to 2.5 mg, my genital area cleared up immediately (within three days). That was approximately eight years ago. It has never returned since, not even for a day.

D.P., Pennsylvania

May/June '99

Exorex

I wanted to share my success with Exorex [tar product] for the scalp. I've been suffering from scalp psoriasis for many years and have tried numerous products, but none have worked this well for me.

K.A.O., Massachusetts

Triamcinolone and Vanicream

I seem to have found something that is helping. It is triamcinolone [topical steroid] and was prescribed to me by a dermatologist from the Mayo Clinic in Scottsdale, AZ. They also told me to use Vanicream, which is an over-the-counter moisturizer. It comes in a tub at most pharmacies and is very inexpensive.

In the 20–30 years I have been suffering from psoriasis, I have tried everything. These two medications seem to work the best for me.
J.R., Michigan

Editor's note: Triamcinolone is a low to medium strength topical steroid medication. For information about Vanicream, contact Pharmaceutical Specialties at (800) 325-8232.

Traditional Chinese medicine

I just read a letter in the March/April 1998 issue of the NPF *Bulletin* from S.D. in Illinois, who stated that her psoriasis cleared after only five treatments of acupuncture. I would like to report a similar experience. I didn't go to a chiropractor, though. I went to a traditional Chinese doctor (a very wonderful lady, who I just love). She began acupuncture treatments once a week and gave me Chinese herbs and an herbal cream. She also suggested a change in my diet—less dairy products, sugar, red meat and fried food.

My skin, scalp and nails have completely cleared in about six weeks. Also, acne that I had on my face and back has cleared. If this wasn't good enough, I've also lost weight and feel so much better.
L.T., Illinois

Anthralin, UVB

I have found that the most effective treatment (and I've tried just about all of them) is anthralin [prescription product], at 4% strength level. I wash it off with a

neutralizing agent after about 35 minutes. This, in combination with UVB lights, seems to clear my skin if I am willing to follow this treatment religiously for about two to three weeks. Your dermatologist might be able to formulate this for you, as does mine. It's messy, time consuming and expensive (usually health plans view it as a specialty item and will not reimburse you for it). The good part is that if it works once, it will continue to work when you need it and doesn't cause a rebound reaction, even though the psoriasis will eventually return.
J.P.S., *New York*

Accutane

I am 52 years old and have had psoriasis for six years. I started with methotrexate, then moved on to Tegison, Soriatane and now Accutane [oral prescription drugs]. The methotrexate, Tegison and Soriatane were devastating to my body. I was always tired and sore and could not get enough sleep. I lost hair on my legs and some on my head. My libido was gone, and it was a very bad experience.

My doctor suggested Accutane, and it has almost cleared my psoriasis. I still have to use ointment around my ears and in my ears, but it has given me new life. Accutane is used primarily for acne and the doctor explained that it helps in about 50 percent of her patients.
M.L., *Texas*

Buttermilk foot soak

A year ago I made a trip to Finland and while in the Helsinki airport, I talked to a dermatologist from the University of Helsinki. She informed me that they had some good results with buttermilk for pustular psoriasis, the type I have. She told me to soak my feet in warm buttermilk for 20 minutes to a half an hour, pat the excess off and encase each foot in a plastic bag and loose socks. She said to only remove and wash in the morning.

After the first "soak," my feet were so different—no burning or swelling. Since then, I have soaked my feet in one pint of buttermilk twice a week and also have been drinking eight ounces of buttermilk every day. After a year and two months, my feet have been really good, though I still bear the marks of broken pustules. But, I have no pain or swelling. I am 81 years old and have been unable to walk normally for more than 20 years. Now I am like a different person, and I think the buttermilk has helped.

M.S., Michigan

Cod liver oil

I want to thank profusely W.P.O. of California ("It Works for Me," Nov/Dec 1998 **Bulletin**) for his suggestion to take cod liver oil for psoriasis. After two short bouts of methotrexate (which did clear it up for about two weeks) prescribed by a dermatologist who uses it only as a last resort, I started to ingest the cod liver oil with a slight mint flavor. It is relatively cheap compared to the topicals.

The results were especially noticeable on my feet. I used to get plaques as large as quarters on them. Mine cleared up in about the same three weeks noted by W.P.O. No longer do I snow all over the house or leave a trail of white wherever I go. I have also virtually eliminated the use of the topicals that I used to apply in the morning and prior to going to bed in the evening. I still use them, but very sparingly since the advent of the cod liver oil.

P.J.K., New Jersey

July/August '99

Vegetarian diet

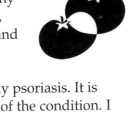

I became a vegetarian about 13 years ago and cut out sugar, in all its forms, severely restricted my refined carbohydrates (and unrefined like potatoes), eliminated all alcohol from my life and started doing one hour of exercise a day. Some or all of these factors, I believe, have virtually eliminated my psoriasis. It is not the natural waxing and waning of the condition. I have been free from "The Heartache" for about five years.

G.S., *California*

Vaseline Intensive Care Lotion

Today, I have a small psoriasis lesion on my right thigh. Last January, I had it all over my body and the doctor prescribed Lac-Hydrin and a tar ointment mixture. This helped me temporarily, and then it would flare up again full-blown.

Then the doctor prescribed pure Vaseline. My skin condition improved. Each evening I would rub my entire body with Vaseline but that would make my pajamas a bit sticky. So I experimented with Extra Strength 12-hour formula Vaseline Intensive Care Lotion. This stopped the itch and the psoriasis lesions. I take a luke warm shower every other night for about five to ten minutes using Dove soap for sensitive skin. After the shower I use the Vaseline lotion.

H.W.L., *Pennsylvania*

Citrus fruit

This worked for my psoriatic arthritis. I had several joints involved for three or more years. The

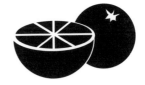

---

injured joints became sausages, and the pain was intense. I read some books on arthritis and stopped eating fruit for a while. Then I narrowed it down to citrus fruits. For six years now I have been pain free, and my joints look and feel normal with a minor amount of stiffness. I even went through a severe skin flare without the arthritis coming back.
A.T., California

Tea tree shampoo
I have been using Paul Mitchell Tea Tree Special Shampoo for about one year and no longer have scalp psoriasis. I recommended it to several friends and they got the same results.
C.G., Kentucky

ZNP soap
I read about ZNP Bar [zinc pyrithione soap] in the *Bulletin*. It has done an incredible job of clearing my scalp after three years of trying. It even cleared my face.
S.S., Texas

September/October '99

Fluocinonide
I had an irritating case of psoriasis on my scalp and ears that I put up with for over two years. I finally went to a general practitioner, who recommended applying fluocinonide cream USP 0.05% [prescription topical steroid] to the affected area three times a day. My condition completely cleared up within four days, and although I was told to apply the cream when I had a flare-up, this has never happened.
P.S., Maryland

Methotrexate, diet

I have read many references in alternative medicine sources to the theory that psoriasis is a symptom of digestive problems, which cause toxins to be eliminated through the skin. My personal experience with severe psoriasis for over 40 years is that animal fats, especially butter, cause severe inflammatory pustular outbreaks—sometimes severe enough to cause bleeding lesions that take weeks to heal. Less severe instances behave like a deep burn—raised deep red blotches with a pustular substance under the skin, which gradually dries and peels.

Although methotrexate has allowed me to live a normal life for the last 12 years, I find that avoiding butter, other dairy products, fatty meats, fowl and fish helps me a great deal. My only other problem food is cantaloupe, from which I get the same reaction. Although Topicort [prescription topical steroid] is helpful to me with other types of outbreaks, it is ineffective with this particular reaction (pustular psoriasis).
J.D., California

Capsaicin formula

Hot pepper, or capsaicin, provides an almost instant relief for my infernal itching. A pharmaceutical manufacturer in Florida markets a 16-ounce container of lotion with a pump. I apply the cream on the most troublesome areas first.
E.K., Florida

Balnetar, Exorex and home UVB

I bathe in Balnetar [tar product], using my prescribed home therapy lamp aggressively, and use Exorex Emulsifying Lotion [tar product] followed by their moisturizer. I am happy to report that my palms, elbows, feet and thighs are greatly improved! I still

have a way to go on my lower legs, but everything is better!
B.D., Georgia

Blue Lagoon clinic

I went to Iceland recently and "soaked" in the waters at the "Blue Lagoon," which apparently is a mineral-laden, geo-thermal pool adjacent to an electric generating plant. After soaking in the very buoyant water for about one hour (outdoors in approximately 35 degree weather), rinsing without use of soap and drying, I noticed that my psoriasis had greatly improved to about the status resulting from a week in the Caribbean sunshine and salt water.

When I initially entered the water, I noticed the slight stinging sensation I usually feel when entering salt water. It always abates in a minute or two, but that is the only similarity between ocean bathing and this "Blue Lagoon" experience. If they offered a place to stay, I would seriously consider returning solely for the use of the water. I was very surprised to experience this abatement of my scaling, redness, soreness, etc., from just that short period of time.
C.E.C., New Jersey

Editor's note: For more information contact Blue Lagoon, Ltd., Svartsengi, PO Box 22, 240 Grindavik, Iceland, (354) 426-8800, or find information on the Web at www.bluelagoon.is.

November/December '99

Surgery for psoriatic arthritis

There was a letter in the July/Aug 1998 *Bulletin* regarding curving of toes that happens for some people with psoriatic arthritis. I had the same problem about four years ago. My toes, with the exception of my big toes, curved under to the extent that I could hardly walk. My doctor removed some bone in the first joint of all eight toes and inserted pins. This was done in one day of surgery.

Following the operation, I could walk using post-op shoes and do normal things like going to work, driving a car, etc. After about 12 days, my doctor removed the pins from the toes and I could put on shoes. I have not had any problems since then and can walk normally.

R.E.G., *Texas*

Enbrel

I have been using Enbrel [prescription product] for severe psoriatic arthritis for two months now and am so excited about the results that I wanted to pass it on to the NPF.

I am a 62-year-old female. For 30 plus years I have taken methotrexate even though it makes me very nauseated. I have taken tablets and for the last two years, I was getting injections once a week.

My dermatologist told me about Enbrel, and I gave it a try. I give myself two shots a week, and I was able to tell after about four shots that this was going to be a new life for me. I am able to do things that I had not been able to do for 15 years (like get up off of the floor without using my arms to pull myself up because the muscles and ligaments in my legs were so affected.)

If I give myself the shot at night, I feel no side effects. In the daytime, I experienced a tiredness or slight flu-like feeling.

Enbrel, as you know, is very expensive. It is about $125 a shot or $1,000 a month. I haven't had any trouble getting Blue Cross/Blue Shield to cover the expense through its mail-in pharmacy program.

P.W., *via e-mail*

Index

N

O

P

vinegar 66, 92
vinyl occlusion suit 89
Virgin Skin Soap 8
vitamin A 73
vitamin C 71
vitamin D_3 73
vitamin D aloe-based bubble
  bath 36
vitamin E 41, 61, 67, 73, 74
vitamin E cream 72
vitamin E gel 54
vitamin E lotion 80
vitamin E oil 79
Vitamin Skin Supplement
  Formula 426 89
vitamin/mineral supplements
  26

W

warm water 25
warm towel 93
washcloth 24
water 10, 11, 24, 26
water purifier 10
water softening system 19
WD-40 11
weight 4, 27
Wesson Vegetable Oil 72
wet packs 11
*What To Say When You Talk To
  Yourself* 41
wheat berries 45
white potatoes 88
white sock 51
whole wheat 36
witch hazel 17, 23, 75, 83
wooden spoon 25
Working Hands Crème 90
wrap 25

X

X-Seb-T Shampoo 11

Y

yeast 89
yoga 74
yogurt 59, 74

Z

Zest 69
Zila Brace Oral Analgesic Gel
  38
Zilactin-B 38
Zim's Crack Creme 93
zinc oxide 7, 15, 22, 68, 75
zinc pyrithione 94, 100
zinc supplement 41

How to Stay Informed

The best way to live with psoriasis is to be informed. The NPF embraces patient education as its primary mission. In fact, the NPF is a past recipient of the American Academy of Dermatology's Excellence in Education Award for its outstanding performance in this area. The NPF member is the direct beneficiary of that excellence.

If you are not an NPF member, join today. NPF members receive the *Bulletin* six times per year and *Psoriasis Resource* three times per year. Membership is a yearly contribution in any amount. For a free packet of information about psoriasis and membership in the NPF, please call (800) 723-9166.

Other educational booklets available from the National Psoriasis Foundation . . .

- Anthralin
- Conception, Pregnancy & Psoriasis
- Cosmetic Cover-Ups
- Cyclosporine (Neoral)
- Genital Psoriasis
- Home Phototherapy
- Methotrexate (MTX)
- Oral Retinoid Therapy (Soriatane)
- Overview of Psoriasis Treatments
- Psoriatic Arthritis
- Psoriasis: How It Makes You Feel
- Psoriasis Research
- Psoriasis on Specific Skin Sites
     (Nails, Ears, Eyelids, Face, Mouth & Lips, Hands & Feet)
- PUVA
- Scalp Psoriasis
- Specific Forms of Psoriasis (Pustular, Guttate, Inverse, Erythrodermic)
- Steroids
- Sunlight & Psoriasis
- Tar
- Things To Consider: Talking with your physician; making treatment decisions; and knowing your rights as a patient
- Topical Retinoid Therapy (Tazorac®)
- Topical Vitamin D_3 (Dovonex)
- UVB
- Young People & Psoriasis
- Your Diet & Psoriasis